CANNABIS CONVERSATIONS

From Confusion to Clarity

32 Leading Experts Share Their Wisdom, Insight & Knowledge About Cannabis & CBD

CYNTHIA DOUGHERTY, PH.D.

ISBN: 978-0-578-67402-5

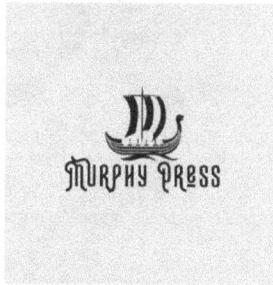

MURPHY PRESS

This book is not intended as a substitute for the medical advice of physicians. The reader should regularly consult a physician in matters relating to his/her health, and particularly with respect to symptoms that may require diagnosis or medical attention.

While the author has made every effort to provide accurate website addresses and other information at the time of publication, neither the publisher nor the author assumes any responsibility for errors or changes that occur after publication. Further, the publisher does not have any control over and does not assume any responsibility for author or third-party websites or their content.

Acknowledgements

This book was assembled as a labor of love. It was a journey of discovery, research, frustration, personal growth, wellness, excitement, and change. I want to express my deepest and most loving gratitude to all of those who have supported, loved, inspired, and supplied me with knowledge and patience. Once again, I left my comfort zone and moved back to Miami to write and gather information. Lessons were learned, all directing me to Self. Life is about finding your mission. Once it's found, the powers that be will guide you through it.

I am very grateful to my children Morgan and Shelby! I love you so much. You have faith in me at times when I question myself. You both are always there cheering me on! For that, I can't thank you enough. I thank my sister Colleen, who thinks that I rock! My mother Ruth for her support. My tribe members, Gina, Janet, Judi, Melanie Fraley, Theresa Marie, Elise, Elizabeth of Delray, and the Ritz gang! My soul sisters, Patricia, Vee, Colleen, Nancy Kane, Paula, Lurenda, and Bunny! You all inspired me, pushed me and challenged me to dig deeper. For that, I am eternally grateful. Life is so much better when we are all together. To Tim, Marisol and Christi Powell, you have taught me so much about CBD! Together we are changing so many people's lives through The Greater Self Boxes and Selph Products. So excited about 2020. It's our year to promote wellness and all of the miracles CBD and Nano can provide.

To Gary Rezeppa and his daughter Jen. I love you both for your support and love. You understood my determination and need to see this project through. I am so grateful. Guess what? Next year, there will be Part 2!

Wayne Dyer says, *"Passion is a feeling that tells you: this is the right thing to do. Nothing can stand in my way. It doesn't matter what anyone else says. This feeling is so good that it cannot be ignored. I'm going to follow my bliss and act upon this glorious sensation of joy."*

This quote is significant on many levels and requires changing your thoughts in order to change your life, as Dyer describes. Surrender and taking a leap of faith is our purpose in this life. It's normal to have second thoughts and also to have fear, but it's all part of the journey.

This book was inspired by my best friend, soul mate and extra mom, Gail. She was an extraordinary role model and human being. She loved life and was grateful every day for her life. Cancer could not slow down her passion for starting a new day. She fought hard with courage, determination, and love. Together, we explored the world of Cannabis. Gail encouraged me to spread the word of its effectiveness and healing powers. She encouraged me to write a guide on Cannabis to make is easier for consumers to make the best choice for themselves.

I could not have written and coordinated this book without the help of Michelle Kulp. Michelle, you are a rare find in this world and so talented. Your passion for books and writing is an inspiration to us all. Your book launches and marketing is such a gift. To my amazing editor, lawyer, judge , comedian, and best friend, Lori Brudner Duff, no words can thank you enough or describe how much you lift me up to be a better person. I admire you from afar. Michelle and Lori, we have more books to write and bring forth ahead. To Alex Strathdee, for your endless patience with collecting the chapters and chasing contributors!

To all of the contributors, I am so thankful you took a chance and wrote your chapters. Your expertise and passion for your professions is limitless. You all love the patients and clients and with the purest intentions, change their lives with CBD. It's an honor to know you all. We share such a personal and needed message about the effectiveness of Cannabis. Together, we can eliminate the stigma and provide the pubic with unbiased research and experiences as well as the importance of looking beyond a label, knowing how products are made, and the important differences that impact your health. Let us be your guide dogs and find the best made products for you!

I hope this inspires you to share the knowledge of CBD with someone who has pain in their lives. Whether it's physical or emotional, or even sleeping issues, it's a game changer!

Table of Contents

Foreword

For change in our world, there has to be those that continuously speak up and show up—the ones that continuously share their story, their truth of this plant. Dr. Cynthia Dougherty is a truth seeker, a motivator, and a trailblazer for all those looking for a seat at the table. As the founder of the Women of Cannabis Conference, I have met women from across the globe. The common mission for all of us is to unleash the stigma, myths, and harsh politics surrounding the Cannabis plant.

Dr. Cynthia has compiled an outstanding list of industry trailblazers that are paving the way for the rest of us! I wish there was a book like this when I decided to dive into the "wild, wild, west of weed." The insider information that is shared is an invaluable source for your Cannabis insights. She did a great job researching and finding those that have real experiences and expertise!

There is such a need in this budding industry to join forces together! We need to hold ourselves accountable at a higher level because we are the foundation to a brand new industry! We are creating the future that will heal the world, but we cannot do it alone. We cannot do it if we do not rise to the occasion and work together on this mission. When we have one common goal, we can achieve anything. It is time that we start the conversation and lift each other up!

This book aligns with our vision so very well! The first step to changing the minds of others is to start the conversation. *Cannabis Conversations* will pique your interest to join our mission in saving the world through Cannabis. It all starts with a conversation!

Stacy Thompson

Founder
Women of Cannabis Conference
Director of Field Development
Simple Changes
www.womenofCannabisconference.com
www.scdso.com

Dedication

To Beverly Gail Privette, Patricia San Pedro,
Judi B Amick, Laura Marshall, Janet Selway,
Dr. Gary Ruben, Cindy Papale-Hammontree,
Bella Rezeppa, and other Cancer Warriors
around the world

"If you change the way you look at things, the things you look at change."

—Dr. Wayne Dyer

"Have within you an imaginary candle flame that burns brightly regardless of what goes before you. Let this inner flame represent for you the idea that you are capable of manifesting miracles in your life."

— Dr. Wayne Dyer

"I've learned that no matter what happens, or how bad it seems today, life does go on, and it will be better tomorrow."

— Maya Angelou

"To develop courage you have to start developing courage as you do any other muscle. You have to start with small things and build it up."

— Maya Angelou

DISCLAIMERS

This book is not a replacement for medical advice from a healthcare professional. The author, publisher, and contributors do not dispense medical advice or prescribe the use of any technique as a form of treatment for physical, emotional, or medical concerns. You should seek the independent advice of a physician. Application of the information described in this book is undertaken at the reader's risk, with no liability to the author, publisher, or contributors. The contents of this book are for educational and informational purposes only. Readers with medical concerns should consult with a healthcare professional. Readers with psychological concerns should consult with a mental health professional.

IMPORTANT FDA DISCLAIMER: The statements made regarding CBD or any Cannabis-related products have not been evaluated by the Food and Drug Administration (FDA). The efficacy of these products has not been confirmed by FDA-approved research. CBD products are not intended to diagnose, treat, cure, or prevent any disease. All information presented here is not meant to substitute for or give an alternative to information from health care practitioners. Please consult your healthcare professional about potential interactions or other possible complications before using any product. The Federal Food, Drug, and Cosmetic Act requires this notice.

An Introduction to Cannabis

There are so many misunderstandings about Cannabis, especially CBD. We want to provide a guide for consumers to understand the exploding CBD market and help weed (ha!) through the thousands of products available. Determining which product is the best for you can be overwhelming. For me, it's like going to The Cheesecake Factory and trying to pick just one item from the thirty-page menu.

I only recently became interested in Cannabis and related products. I lived a very sheltered life when I was young. I went to an all-girls' Catholic school, and I wasn't exposed to marijuana at all when I was there. In college, I saw it only from a distance. I didn't consider it a part of my life until my mother was diagnosed with cancer.

My mother developed a cough. She told us not to worry about it. It was just allergies. It was the humidity. We bought her a humidifier and an air purifier for her room. We worried about respiratory issues because we knew we were exposed to a lot of carcinogens after our house caught fire during the wildfires in California many years ago. We tried hard to buy into her, "don't worry" attitude, but the cough worsened as the years went by.

It took threats of bodily harm to get her to go back to the doctor. He gave her another course of antibiotics but didn't take any x-rays or scans. After three weeks with no improvement, she went back. He gave her more antibiotics and a course of steroids. Tick tock, tick tock. Time was a-wasting! Her cough improved a little bit after the steroids, but it was still there. We went back to the doctor. Finally, he ordered imaging.

Mom was in no rush to give us bad news. She waited until after the holidays to share the results. I looked at the copies of the scans the doctor had given her. It looked like someone had shaken a snow globe inside of her chest. There were several small confetti-type circles all over her lungs.

If only that were the worst of it. The cancer had begun in her stomach and then spread into her lungs and intestines. I had been through this before. I had lost a friend before at the age of 48. She experienced the same symptoms. She had a cough and no history of smoking. They kept giving her antibiotics and steroids. No other testing or scans for months. She died two months later.

My mother lingered a whole lot longer than that. She suffered a whole lot longer than that. She had an iron will to live. She never complained, loved life, and was a warrior. She wasn't afraid to die and made the best of every day.

Cancer is a horrible disease, and watching it claim a loved one is a horrible process. It is a never-ending stream of stress, pain, frustration, blood tests, scans, chemo ports, hair loss, isolation, anxiety, and fear. The list of experiences is endless. It's something for the patient to endure, and the caregivers as well. It's excruciating for everyone involved.

I watched a confident, calm, happy, physically strong, mischievous jokester turn into a frail, sad woman who at times suffered panic attacks. One minute she would be fine, and the next she would be crying uncontrollably.

She had stage four cancer and, on a bad day, could not get out of bed. She often suffered from uncontrollable coughing fits. She resisted taking pain meds for as long as she could. As a former ER nurse, she feared a dependency to opiates more than she feared dying. She didn't want to fall or feel groggy. After all, she had to keep her mind sharp for her Friday night bingo games!

Refilling her pain meds required an office visit and a urine test. This seemed ridiculous to me. She was in too much pain to get out of bed. We needed to find an alternative.

I started reading everything I could get my hands on about Cannabis. If it wasn't in print, I would call people or knock on their doors to get answers. I flew to California and Colorado. All along, I was grateful for being able to make her life a little more bearable.

Since the industry was new, and at the time, half of it was underground, trying to understand the whole concept of Cannabis as a consumer was overwhelming, confusing, and surprising to me. I reached out to friends. The topic felt almost secretive. Many people were using Cannabis products but somehow felt like there was a stigma attached to them. They worried that others would judge them. As I disrobed my need for my mother, the doors flew open. People came out of the woodwork, telling their stories and offering help and recommendations.

If you know me, you know that this led to a million different questions. Where can you buy Cannabis? What is CBD? What is THC? Is it legal? Can I mail it? Can I take it on a plane? Is it toxic? Can you overdose? Can it be combined with other drugs? What if you don't have time to apply for a medical card? What is the best way to use CBD? Are all CBD products the same? What are the side effects? How do you know which product is the best for you? Can it affect your security clearance? Will it show up on a drug test?

The questions were endless. But so were the answers.

One step at a time, I brought her different types of CBD and THC products to try. We were in this together. She was so much happier. Her mood changed. I witnessed the anxiety associated with cancer lessen. Her appetite increased, and she slept like a log. Once she opened up about her discovery, the other women in her building showed her their stash! How sad – they all felt scared and worried they would be judged, but they all loved their products. Wouldn't it have been better if they had been able to tell others how much these products had helped them? They all felt better in so many ways and they could have helped others feel better, too.

After my mother passed away, I decided I wanted to share this gift with as many people as I could. I made the decision to become an advocate and educator of Cannabis. It was the best gift I could offer her during the most painful time in her life. As a Master Mind Performance Coach, a Neuropsychologist, and Human Development Specialist, I have a particularized understanding of the wellness, psychological, and physiological aspects of Cannabis. I want to use this book to help people get the most out of their Cannabis experiences.

As consumers, we have so many questions, and not enough answers. I always recommend consulting with a healthcare professional who is knowledgeable about CBD before adding it to your life and your other medications. Get as much information as you can before making a decision about what is right for you.

Not all CBD products are the same. Select CBD products based on your individual needs. When my Mom was suffering with cancer, I looked for comfort for her pain. What was the easiest method that would work for her and her individual needs? There is no one-size-fits-all solution for any given condition. What works for me might not work for you.

Two people with similar diagnoses and conditions can have completely different reactions to CBD delivery methods and dosages. In writing this book, I asked as many people as I could find about their experiences with CBD to learn what they tried, how it worked for them, and their ultimate recommendations.

Cannabinoids – despite consistency in dose, delivery method, and cannabinoid – do not affect each person in the same way. Scientists are still researching what makes these differences. Until the results of these investigations are available, you have to do your own experimentation when you start taking CBD.

Gradually increase the dosage in small increments. If, after taking the lower dosage, you don't begin to see results within a few days, increase the dosage and try the higher dosage for a few days. CBD oil takes time to build up in your system before you see results, and its effects are often more subtle than you might expect. People who have experienced the instant high of the THC in marijuana might be surprised by how subtle the effects of CBD are. It might take a few days before you notice any particular changes in your emotional state.

It's important that you don't rush to increase the dosage until you've given it enough time to build up in your system. Whatever your total dose is, break it down into smaller doses throughout the day. For example, if your plan is to take 500 mg, don't take a single 500 mg dose. Take five 100 mg doses throughout the day, or something similar. While it is safe to take CBD in large doses, taking too much of it at one time could cause you to lose some of its efficacy. It's best to introduce it into your system in smaller increments to allow your body to better absorb the CBD and increase its efficacy at the same time.

Pay attention to and be particularly observant of your own self to notice the changes CBD can have. The changes are not always obvious, but they can be. Sublingual (under the tongue) products used for anxiety relief can provide quick benefits.

It can be helpful to layer delivery products. CBD can be introduced into your system in many ways:

- via edibles
- sublingually
- via oils in your beverages
- in lotions, creams, tinctures, suppositories
- via inhalation

Using various forms of CBD can be helpful to gain maximum benefits.

CBD can be "biphasic" meaning that it can have a different effect depending on the dose that you take. For example, a small amount of CBD can have a stimulating effect and help you focus and keep your attention. If you take a large amount of CBD, the effect can be sedating. The trick is to find the sweet spot that works for you. It's a curve, and the size and slope of the curve depends on the individual. What works for one person can be a disaster for another person, and vice versa. A dose that helps one person focus may make another person's eyelids droop. Taking too much may cause the opposite problem. While a low dose may mellow your mood, a high dose may amplify anxiety. Most experts (including me) will tell you to, "start low and go slow." That's the safest and most effective route to finding that sweet spot. Don't worry if you don't see results immediately. That's just your body getting used to CBD.

Common Side Effects

One of the first questions people ask about CBD is, "What are the side effects?" Because it is such a close cousin to marijuana, people wonder if it will make them high or intoxicated. The good news is that it won't! That isn't to say that there aren't any side effects, though most people won't experience any.

The most common side effects of CBD are

- Fatigue
- Diarrhea
- Changes in appetite

These changes are not generally significant. If they are, stop taking CBD and contact your healthcare provider.

Less common side effects are:

- Dry mouth
- Dizziness or faintness
- Increased anxiety

If you experience increased anxiety, it may be a sign that you are taking too much. If cutting back on CBD does not reduce the anxiety, your system may not be able to tolerate even small doses of CBD. This is rare, but it does happen.

CBD can interact with other drugs that you are taking. It can also make certain medical conditions, like glaucoma, worse. CBD is a P450 inhibitor, just like grapefruit. P450 is the name of a group of enzymes that help break down drugs in your body to make them work properly. If the P450 enzymes are inhibited, that is, if they can't do their job, then the drugs don't break down and they collect in your liver. That can be dangerous. A good rule of thumb is that if grapefruit would interfere with your medications, then CBD will, too. If you are taking over-the-counter or prescription medications, always check with your prescribing doctor and/or a qualified pharmacist before you start taking CBD.

Like everything else, if you have any questions about what is going on with your body, be sure to talk to a healthcare professional who is familiar with cannabinoid medicine before taking CBD.

What is the difference between CBD and Marijuana?

CBD comes from hemp, which is a very close relative of marijuana. The plants look very similar and share many of the same properties. The main difference between the two plants is the presence of THC, or delta-9 transtetrahydrocannibanol (Say that three times fast!). THC is the chemical in marijuana that gets you 'high.' There is some THC in hemp, but in order to be considered hemp, agriculturally and legally, there has to be less than .3% of THC in the plant. In comparison, marijuana used for intoxication purposes will have somewhere around 20% of THC—more than 60 times more THC.

There has been a lot of debate in the U.S. House of Representatives and Senate about how to distinguish the useful, non-intoxicating hemp from marijuana, and how to regulate the agricultural product without running afoul of the Controlled Substances Act. Finally, in the 2018 Farm Bill, an agreement was reached in principle. CBD can now be sold in US states that have approved medical marijuana or have sanctioned marijuana for adult consumption. This explains the recent explosion of CBD retail outlets and the visibility of CBD products in health food stores.

CBD Delivery Methods

When you are choosing your delivery method, be aware of bioavailability. Bioavailability is how much of a specific compound – in this case, CBD –is available for your body to use. The more bioavailability, the more likelihood that the compound is used by your body. Everything that you put in your body – nutrients in foods and supplements, over-the-counter and prescription medications, and things like Cannabis in all of its forms – have a certain level of bioavailability.

The level of bioavailability is different for each person. The same product, the same apple, the same Vitamin C supplement, chocolate cake, whatever it is, is going to have a different bioavailability depending on the individual. There is no universal way to measure it. Multiple factors contribute to bioavailability, like stomach acid (gastric pH), body chemistry, metabolism, gender, age, diet, and other environmental factors.

Let's get a quick rundown of some of the most common delivery methods and some of the advantages of each. We'll go over them in more detail later in this book.

Oral

Oral products go through the digestive system before making it into the bloodstream. Products that are taken under the tongue (sublingual products) have high bioavailability because they can be absorbed directly into the blood vessels underneath the thin skin beneath your tongue before you swallow them. You can find oral products in:

- Capsules and gel caps
- Edibles (like gummies)
- Beverages
- Tinctures (in oil or alcohol bases)
- Fiber

Vaporized and Nebulized Products

Vaporized and nebulized CBD products are effective almost immediately, but the effects fade almost as quickly. They don't last nearly as long as those of other delivery systems. You can find them in hemp flower oil for vaporizers and water for nebulizers, and nasal sprays.

Suppositories

Because suppositories are absorbed directly into the bloodstream without being broken down by stomach acids, they have high bioavailability. They work for any issue that CBD can treat.

Transdermal

Topicals, such as balms, salves, lotions, shampoos, bath bombs, face and beauty products, creams, gel, and patches are available. They are for topical use only. They can be effective for localized pain but may not be as bioavailable for other conditions.

Inhalers

Smoking or vaporizing CBD is a very common choice. When you smoke CBD oil, it is easy to manage your dose, so you know exactly how much you are consuming. However, smoking has the very negative side effect of irritating your throat and lungs, which can lead to more problems later. Don't solve one problem just to create another one down the line.

Vaping CBD is one of the most popular ways of getting it into your system, and it may have the same benefits of smoking CBD without the negative side effects.

What Can and Can't Cannabis Do?

Like everything else in life, there are a lot of misconceptions about Cannabis. Just to name a few, some people believe that it can cure anything. I've heard people say that CBD works best without THC. There's a common misconception that all CBD products are the same. Some people believe that THC is the bad cannabinoid and CBD is the good cannabinoid, or that THC is recreational and CBD is medicinal. Some people believe that CBD is sedating and makes you sleepy, or that it is only safe for adults. There is a misbelief that hemp and marijuana are the same plant instead of cousins. People also tend to think that CBD comes from marijuana instead of hemp.

Side effects from CBD are rare, but they do occur. Most common side effects are mild and include decreased appetite, GI upset, diarrhea, and nausea. These side effects go away as soon as you stop consuming CBD, and they might go away if you decrease your dosage.

While Cannabis can't cure every disease, it can help quite a bit with some common and not-so-common diseases. Its use in helping to control seizures in epilepsy and other seizure-related disorders is legendary. THC is a known appetite stimulant and has proven invaluable in helping chemotherapy patients maintain their weight

My son was diagnosed with Ehlers-Danlos Syndrome, which is a relatively rare disorder (fewer than 200,000 cases per year are diagnosed) that affects the connective tissues in the body, mostly the skin, joints, and blood vessels. As you age, it weakens the connective tissues. In my son's case, his joints are mainly affected, and he is starting to experience daily pain. Several doctors have recommended pain meds on the bad days. This was not an option for him.

We began experimenting with CBD oils, topicals, patches, and vape products. It was life changing for him. He carries a pain stick and salve with him during the day at school and work. Depending on the method, his pain will dissipate within 20 minutes. He is now sharing his products with his friends and colleagues at work. He is also a handy and familiar product tester for me, and my business.

I can personally report that my daily use of CBD has helped increase focus, reduce stress, and increase stamina.

It's a new industry, and as the industry grows, there will be improvements and enhancements in CBD and other Cannabis products. Traditional drug companies will launch research studies, increasing our understanding of what it can and cannot do and in what ways. New products will be introduced on the market as our knowledge increases.

The more it becomes commercially available and the more it is marketed in traditional ways, the less stigma will be attached to it. The general population will discover new ways to make Cannabis a part of their lives for social purposes and wellness.

As this occurs, the U.S. federal government is going to have to get on board and establish policies that not only allow Cannabis to be legalized nationwide but create consistent regulation. Consistent regulation will benefit consumers, as you will be able to look at a label and know that there are enforceable rules governing what is listed on the packaging.

I foresee Cannabis as a real solution to the opioid crisis. With a viable alternative to opioids as a relief for suffering, the addictions won't happen, overdosing won't occur, and there won't be deaths.

CBD DOSAGE AND METHODOLOGY

CBD products are required to include serving size and nutritional information on the food labels, but that information is not the same as dosage information, and you shouldn't confuse the two. The information on those labels is more related to nutrition and calories than it is to CBD efficacy. It is an educated guess, but it may be unrelated to what works for you.

Unlike other over-the-counter medications like Ibuprofen or Acetaminophen where the recommended dosage is clearly marked on the label, CBD oil is not that easy. The results of what you take will be based on your individual receptors within your body. What dosage may work for one person may not work at all for you or may be far too much for you. So, how do you figure it out?

If you're not familiar with vaping, you can start with one of the more popular options, CBD Vape-Oil. This contains somewhere between 50 and 100 milligrams of cannabidiol, the active substance, in each dose. Many vape starter kits can help you get the hang of it without much effort. Vape cartridges come in a variety of flavors, including natural flavors. Once you feel comfortable using it, then you can move on to some of the stronger doses, which will max out at 200 mg.

Vaping is a safer alternative to smoking with the same effects in terms of bioavailability and speed of delivery. Because the vaporized CBD oil goes directly into the blood circulation through the lungs, the CBD gets to work immediately. Of course, the flip side is also true – because it gets to work quickly, it also wears off quickly. The effects don't last as long as other methods like sublingual.

Many people don't feel comfortable with vaping for a variety of reasons. People with respiratory issues, especially, may want to avoid this. Even if you don't mind vaping or find vaping relaxing, you may want to supplement vaping with a longer lasting method of introducing CBD to your body.

CBD concentrates are another option, especially if you're looking for stronger results. Keep in mind that CBD concentrates are *concentrated* which means they can hold as much as ten times more cannabinoid than any other product out there. So, be careful! They're easy to calculate and measure but be aware that you are getting a powerful punch of a dose. Concentrates are popular among people who are busy and don't have a lot of time to wait for the weaker products to take effect.

A CBD tincture is the liquid extract of the Cannabis plant. When you buy a tincture, it is not a pure CBD oil. It is usually dissolved in alcohol or other substances that could have a less desirable effect on your health. If you're planning on using a tincture, it is important that you read the labels carefully and use a reputable brand to ensure ingredients not listed on the label have not been added. It is imperative to know exactly what you are getting, and any possible side effects that other substances might cause. Consider that a certain amount of rodent hair is acceptable in commercially produced peanut butter, but you won't find it on the label[1].

Tinctures generally have a high dosage of CBD oil in them and, as a result, can have a strong effect when taken. Because they are mixed with other products like alcohol, vegetable glycerin, or flavorings, you are getting a diluted form of the product.

Tinctures can be found in the form of sprays or drops. The concentration is usually anywhere from 100 mg to 500 mg per dose. To take the drops, place them under your tongue (sublingually) and hold them there for at least 30 seconds before swallowing. The advantage to doing this is that rather than passing through your entire digestive system, the CBD gets absorbed directly into your bloodstream through the blood vessels underneath your tongue, increasing their bioavailability. The longer

---

[1] This is disgusting, but true. https://www.cbsnews.com/pictures/11-revolting-things-government-lets-in-your-food/4/

you can hold the drops there without swallowing, the greater the effect will be.

Tinctures are generally one of the purest forms of CBD oil that you can find. If done correctly, there is no extra processing of the oil. You can find some brands that offer added flavors, which might make the oil a little easier to take because it will mask the oil's unique taste. Without any flavoring, CBD oil has a nutty and earthy taste. It's like vegetables – some people are going to like it, and some people are going to hate it.

If you use the sublingual method, you will notice the effects within about ten to fifteen minutes, and the effects should last about three hours. Obviously, this will vary from person to person, but on average, this is what you should expect.

Edibles are just what they sounds like – gummies, chocolate bars, baked goods, lozenges, drinks, and the like, all made with CBD oil as an ingredient. They have varying amounts of CBD oil in them, so you should read the labels carefully. Because edibles need to pass through the digestive system, they take a little longer to have an effect, but otherwise should work the way tinctures do.

You can find edibles in almost any form. Beware, though, because it is sometimes difficult to know how much CBD you are taking in an edible. They may take up to two hours to take effect, so people have a tendency to think they aren't working and consume more. The good news is that they can last longer in your system. Some people like edibles because of the portability and convenience. No one thinks much of you unwrapping a piece of candy and popping it in your mouth. This may make them more 'work-friendly' than other options like swallowing pills or vaping.

Topicals help soothe physical discomfort and boost the body's natural ability to heal. One of the biggest advantages to using the topicals is that the skin naturally absorbs the oils very quickly and it can go to work on the affected area almost immediately. Although they do work well, they are not as strong as the treatments that can be ingested or inhaled, and do not come in high dosages. This means that the results will be both temporary and limited, and you may need to reapply them frequently for maximum effect. There's nothing wrong with this health-wise, but it can be inconvenient and expensive.

Topicals come in the form of lotions, creams, balms, salves, ointments, and oils. Added ingredients make all the difference. Think about the products that you use for your skin that don't have CBD in them. They feature a variety of skin-healing ingredients, as well as fragrances and other fillers, some good, some bad. The same is true for pain relief and muscle relaxation products. Some products contain aloe for inflamed skin, salves with peppermint oil for sore muscles, and massage creams with essential oils, like lavender, for relaxation.

There are ingredients you may want to avoid. According to the Environmental Working Group, look for the following in the list of ingredients and avoid them when you can:

- BHA & BHT
- Formaldehyde
- Artificial fragrances
- Mineral oil
- Parabens
- Phthalates
- Polyethylene and PEGs
- Propylene glycol
- Retinyl Palmitate, retinyl acetate, retinoic acid, and retinol
- Siloxanes
- Sodium lauryl sulfate and sodium laureth sulfate
- Synthetic colors
- Triclosan and triclocarbon
- Toluene

When you are picking out a topical product, you should look for words like "encapsulation," "nano-technology," and "micellization." These words are good indicators that the CBD product is processed in a way that will allow it to carry through the layers of your skin to provide relief.

Only use the topical CBD product when you need it, and only use it where you need it. If your hamstring is sore, don't cover your entire leg with it, otherwise you will waste it. It can take up to fifteen minutes to take effect, but the effects should last as long as if you were ingesting the oil.

A transdermal patch is applied to your skin and delivers the cannabinoid gradually to your body over a four to six hour period. The patch looks similar to a large adhesive bandage, but you can put it somewhere on your body under your clothes where it can't be seen. Be sure to put it on a part of your body where there are a lot of veins close to the surface. Many people put them on their upper arm, chest, or stomach. Beware – if you stick the patch on your body where there is hair, the hair may interfere with the ability of the patch to do its work. So, find a place that is relatively hairless or remove the hair from that place before sticking the patch on.

Transdermal patches are particularly useful for sports injuries, menstrual pain, and migraines. They're also good if you have a super busy lifestyle and can't stop what you are doing to take additional doses during the day.

One of the reasons they are very effective is that they avoid metabolism in your liver, improving bioavailability. The slower, more sustained delivery of cannabinoids to tissues also helps their effectiveness over time.

CBD sprays have the weakest concentration of CBD oil and have a tendency to be inconsistent. Generally, they only contain one to three milligrams of CBD, which isn't very much compared to other products. They will kick in quickly – usually within ten minutes – but don't last long; only about an hour or two.

Capsules are another option that are a great choice if your plan is to take a daily supplement. Capsules are tasteless and easy to consume. However, because capsules have to pass through the digestive tract, they can lose some bioavailability in the process. To help avoid this, look for capsules that are "enteric-coated." This will help them prevent breakdown in the stomach and help protect the CBD from damage by stomach acids.

One major advantage to capsules is the clarity of dosing. You know exactly what you are getting in each pill. It's already filled, so you know what it is and it is easier to monitor your dose. The downside of that is that if you want to change your dose, it can be difficult. You can't cut a capsule in half, because it is filled with liquid. The capsules are better when you have figured out what your optimal dosage is; until then, use a more flexible form of CBD, like tinctures. Then, once you know exactly how much to take, you can switch to the capsules. If you want to scale up your dose, you can take your regular capsules, and add a drop or two of the tinctures or another product.

When you are using the capsules, remember to stay hydrated to achieve the desired results.

Capsules can take a while before you feel the results. Since they have to be broken down by your digestive tract, it can be between a half an hour and two hours before you feel the effects.

WHAT YOU SEE IS WHAT YOU GET

Some reports show that less than half of the CBD products on the market are actually quality products. Naturally, when you are spending your hard-earned money on a product, you want it to be something that is going to work.

Even if the CBD oil itself is high quality, you want to make sure that the oil is blended with quality products, too. You don't want your CBD mixed with dangerous impurities or have it laced with other products that will do more harm than good. Always read the labels.

In this chapter, we're going to take a look at what you'll often find on a CBD product label so you can understand what you're seeing.

You Get What You Pay For

Unfortunately, it isn't possible to get true, functional CBD oil at a very low price. If you find a real bargain, odds are good that it isn't a very high-quality product. Why is that?

For one, the term "hemp oil" can be a bit confusing. There is a difference between whole plant hemp oil and the extract from the hemp flower. Whole plant hemp oil contains various cannabinoids, terpenes, and other plant materials, creating what is called an "entourage effect." For that reason, CBD products that you consume by mouth are generally whole plant hemp oils. CBD isolates are usually used in skincare and beauty products. To make it more confusing, there is the hemp oil that is used in cooking and on salads. This is a completely different product made from a different part of the hemp plant altogether.

A quick visual will not always tell you what you need to know. Some products may look identical but aren't if you look at the details. Look at the volume and concentration. Two tincture bottles may both contain three ounces, but one may have a lot more CBD oil in it. If one bottle is cheaper than the other, check to see if it is a food category of hemp oil designed more for salads than medicinal use. If you are confused, make sure you select whole plant hemp oil or extract for the healing uses discussed in this book.

Your Body is a Temple

Whatever your religion, you wouldn't make an impure offering to your God. Your body is a temple and you need to treat it that way. Only bring the best to the altar in your temple. That goes for your CBD products as well. It is important that your CBD products are free of artificial ingredients, pesticides, and other harmful chemicals.

If you can, make sure that a third-party agency has tested the products you are buying. Ask the merchant you are purchasing your CBD products through to show you a recent certification of analysis. If they can't provide this, ask them why they can't.

Read the Label

The label on your CBD product should conform to the dietary supplement labeling category requirements. It can provide a lot of information if you know what you are looking for. At a minimum, it should tell you:

- The name of the product and the company that manufactured and distributed it
- The type of CBD – whole plant or isolate
- The milligrams of extract in the total product and per serving
- Ingredients listed in descending order of amount
- Directions for use and the recommended dosage

It may also contain more information which can be helpful, such as:

- The source of the plant – organic, sustainable farm, or not
- The strain of the plant
- Basic supplement facts
- Extraction method used
- Good manufacturing practices, or GMP
- Third-party testing verifications

If at all possible, choose an organic product. All forms of Cannabis are bio-accumulators. This means that hemp plants draw toxins from the soil. They are absorbed more into the seed than the flower. When the CBD oil is extracted and concentrated, the toxins will be extracted and concentrated along with the oil. So it is important that you get your oil from plants that were grown on farms that use organic growing practices, free of pesticides and other harmful chemicals, because then there will be fewer toxins absorbed into the plants.

Unfortunately, there is not an agreed-upon definition of "organic." The United States Department of Agriculture (USDA) doesn't have a certification for what is and is not organic Cannabis or hemp, so the term can be used loosely by unscrupulous growers and manufacturers. Do your research on the source so you know what you are getting and whether you are ingesting poisons.

Sometimes, you will find artificial or unnecessary ingredients in your CBD products. CBD works on its own and does not require any chemical fillers, additives, preservatives, or flavors. It's ok to have additives, but make sure they aren't harmful. Check the label to make sure that you don't have any artificial colorings, flavorings, or sweeteners. Also, avoid high-fructose corn syrup, GMOs, and preservatives and thinning agents like propylene glycol.

Not all added ingredients are bad. You may see additional carrier oils or beneficial herbs added to the product you are considering purchasing. It isn't odd to see coconut oil, MCT oil, or hemp seed oil listed on the label. That doesn't mean that this isn't a CBD product, it just means that they are being diluted in those oils. In CBD vape products, you will usually find that either propylene glycol (PG) or vegetable glycerine (VG) is included. CBD vape liquids should not include carrier oils, since vaping additional oils can be harmful to your health.

Because whole plant CBD products are a new category on the market, there is little to no standardization. Hemp can only be grown commercially in a few U.S. states, so much of it is imported from China and Eastern Europe, where standards may not be enforced. Even within the United States, hemp-growing laws are new and vary, so quality control standards across the board may be inconsistent.

That's why you want to look for third-party testing for quality control to better understand what is in the product and its efficacy. The results of that testing won't be on the label; you'll have to ask for the "Certification of Analysis" or the "C of A." The lab testing results will be able to tell you if the product you are getting is free of contaminants like bacteria, fungus, heavy metals, mold, pesticides, and solvents.

When you are reviewing the lab tests, you need to know the batch number and/or the QR code to tie the specific product you are looking at to the testing that was done. It wouldn't do you any good to look at the testing of another batch of CBD. If there is a QR code on the label, you might be able to link directly to the test results with your smartphone or other device.

Even the most reputable of brands can vary between batches. That's normal and understandable when you are dealing with organic products. The terpenes and cannabinoid content can be slightly different due to differences in soil conditions, resulting in the occasional report of different effects being experienced from the same brand of CBD products. Batch testing allows you to see the variation between batches so you can make intelligent, educated decisions on brand choices and purchasing decisions. Once you determine what you like and what works for you, you can make choices based on batches that are particularly high in the micro-ingredients that work best with your particular body chemistry.

Getting CBD oil from hemp isn't a matter of waving a magic wand over the hemp plant and the oil appearing. You can't just squeeze it out like you'd squeeze the juice from a lemon, either. It has to be extracted from the plant. Not all extraction methods are equally good. Avoid methods that use unsafe solvents like butane or hexane, because then you end up with butane or hexane in the final product. Remember: butane is lighter fluid. You wouldn't drink lighter fluid or use it to flavor your brownies. Why would you want it in anything else you are putting in your body?

Unfortunately, a lot of brands use ethanol from GMO corn and hexane in the extraction process. Hexane is a byproduct of gasoline – yes, the same gasoline that you put in your car. It is not safe for human consumption.

Alcohol extraction is the safest and best method of extraction. When done properly and with care, it is harmless and produces the purest CBD oil for human consumption.

CBD labels will provide the name of the manufacturer and/or the distributor of the product. This doesn't always tell you anything on its face, but it does give you useful information. You can research the manufacturer and distributor yourself to determine the reputation and historical reliability of the company. It's also a good idea to look up the company's testing methods to ensure that you will be taking a product that is pure and free of contaminants.

Most labels will give you a suggested serving size, servings per unit, and servings per package. This combination of information will give you an idea of how long the product you are considering will last. For example, if a .5 gram serving is suggested, and the product contains 20 servings, it will last you 20 days if you consume a .5 gram serving per day. However, if you need more or less CBD than is suggested, the package will last you longer or less time. Like everything else, follow the guidance of your CBD-competent health care provider.

You also want to know how much hemp oil is in the product that you are taking and what part of the plant from which the hemp oil was extracted. Like we talked about earlier, whole-plant extract is going to have a much different effect on your body than extract taken solely from the flower.

Naturally, the amount of CBD present in the product is critical information. The amount of CBD present is not the same as the amount of hemp oil. The product may or may not have trace amounts of THC, which may have different effects on your body. If it does contain THC, the potency information should be on the label as well. Using the .5 gram serving example above, there may be 85 mg of CBD in each serving. This would be a beneficial dose for those using CBD for its healing and therapeutic effects. Work with your doctor to determine the right dosage for you based on what you are trying to accomplish. It will vary depending on your personal body chemistry, your particular condition, and the potency in each serving.

While we talked about avoiding artificial sweeteners and flavorings, there is nothing wrong with using natural sweeteners and flavorings. Sometimes the taste of CBD will interfere with your ability to get the most out of the product, and if flavoring it helps, go for it! The flavoring information on the label will help guide you to one that will work best for your tastes.

Some products will list cautions and storage instructions on the labels. Some may suggest refrigeration, while some say you should keep them away from heat, light, and humidity. Some may just have an expiration date, as after a while, like most oils, CBD oil will go rancid.

CBD oil can be full spectrum, broad spectrum, or an isolate, and the label should tell you which one it is. It may not explicitly use those words, but it should have some kind of indicator specific to that brand. Full spectrum products have a wide range of cannabinoids in addition to CBD, most notably trace amounts of THC and other terpenes. Typically, this range is naturally occurring in the strain of hemp. Broad spectrum products have a range of cannabinoids and terpenes, but no THC. Isolates only have CBD.

The bottle size can also tell you a little bit about what you are getting. Usually, CBD comes in 15 ml (.5 ounce), 30 ml (1 ounce) and 100 ml (3.38 ounces) sizes. If you find yourself with a 16 ounce bottle of, "hemp oil," you probably don't have CBD, but the type of hemp oil that is used for salads and that sort of thing. If you tested the hemp oil, it wouldn't have any CBD in it.

Some people get confused and think that the bigger the bottle, the more CBD. While it is true that there is more CBD total, that is only because there is more liquid in the bottle. Each drop has the same strength. It is not more potent or stronger simply because the bottle is bigger. A 30 ml bottle with 1000 mg of CBD has the same potency as a 15 ml bottle with 500 mg of CBD. In both cases, there are 33.3 milligrams of CBD per milliliter. You might need to do some math to make sure, but don't confuse bottle size with strength.

A "drop" is not a universal standard measurement. A drop will be a different size depending upon the size of the dropper. Make sure you look at the serving size when you are reading the label on the bottle. Most droppers will come in .5 or 1 milliliter sizes. If you have a calibrated dropper or one with numbers on the side, it will help you make sure you are getting the right amount of CBD in your dose. If you don't have a calibrated dropper, use an oral syringe to help you get the correct dosage.

The U.S. Food and Drug Administration (FDA) has not approved CBD, so there are no national standards or requirements when it comes to CBD labels. This can be a real problem, so it is important to make sure you are dealing with a reputable manufacturer. Most companies pledge to give their consumers reliable information but not all of them do, and there aren't any regulations to enforce. Some states that have medical or adult use cannabinoid laws may have some enforceable regulations on labeling but most don't, so you're on your own when it comes to doing research. The industry is self-regulated, and some companies are more ethical than others. Don't forget this – the smiling, sincere face of the salesperson should not substitute for your own legwork.

THC-specific labelling

If you are in a state that allows medical THC or marijuana usage, the labeling should tell you how much THC is in the product. In that case, you want to look at the total THC (or THC maximum) that is available for use. This will give you a good idea of the total psychoactivity of the strain. High THC strains typically have around 18-20% of THC.

When you are looking at edibles, the amount of THC is more often represented in milligrams rather than percentages. In some states, you can find edibles with a whopping 100 or more milligrams. If you are looking for a powerful high, 20 milligrams is considered a large dose, so 100 milligrams is five times that! Whoa.

In products containing THC, you can usually visit the testing lab website to get more information. When you do, you might find out more information about the residual solvents. You also might get information about terpenes. Terpenes are a class of organic compounds created by plants and are a large component of many essential oils. The different terpenes in your product can affect the flavor and aroma and add depth to the psychoactivity of the THC. They may also enhance the medical benefits of the product you are using.

HOW DOES CANNABIS WORK?

We know that CBD is a regulator of many of our body functions. It contributes to wellness and assists with the healing of many health conditions. When you think about it, it's amazing that one single plant contains such a wide variety of medicinal molecules that so widely influence human homeostasis and balance, the powerful connections within all cells that promotes healing, and the optimal function of our organs and organ systems.

Knowing anecdotally how well it works for our bodies and how much more there is to learn is frustrating. There are so many regulatory obstacles that are slowing down scientists. There is only so much research we can do right now on the influences of cannabinoids on the endocannabinoid system in our bodies and how it affects our brain and our bodies, let alone the quality of our lives.

That isn't to say that we don't know anything. There is a good bit that we do know. Cannabidiol, or CBD, is a non-psychoactive chemical produced by the Cannabis plant. It is non-addictive and non-toxic. It's extracted from the plant and then made into a concentrate. Depending on your age and needs, it can treat anything from skin issues to cancer. Adults can tolerate high doses with no risk of overdose or major adverse effects on their heart rate or blood pressure.

Our bodies naturally have an endocannabinoid system, also known as an ECS. The ECS involves a group of both receptors and molecules. It's made up of neural pathways, neurons, receptors, signaling molecules, and enzymes. Our ECS is a major signaling network system. It is one of the rulers of neurotransmission and pain signaling to the brain. That's why CBD works so well in controlling pain.

The ECS is present throughout our bodies just like our nervous system is present throughout our bodies. It's in charge of governing neurotransmission and neuron communication. Our nerves have to communicate with each other, and our ECS helps them do it. Therefore, our ECS is a major influencer over our brains in terms of:

- Memory
- Mood
- Perception
- Cognition
- Motor Functioning
- Emotions
- Rewards
- Anti-inflammation

As if that weren't enough, the ECS also manages the mechanisms of our brain development and protection. It's a regulator of physiological effects, health, wellness, and homeostasis. This means it helps ensure that your body is working well and you have an internal balance. It makes sure you are feeling good as opposed to experiencing that "off-kilter" feeling. Your nervous system, digestion, respiration, and reproductive system are all happy. When they are happy, you are happy.

The ECS itself is comprised of a group of molecules called endocannabinoids and receptors called endocannabinoid receptors. The first system consists of CB1 receptors (cannabinoid receptor 1) which are mostly found in the brain. Things like motor skills, sleep, emotions, pain, brain development, addictive behaviors, learning, and nausea are affected by CB1. It is mostly expressed in the central nervous system, including the hippocampus, cerebral cortex, cerebellum, basal ganglia, hypothalamus, and amygdala. It can be found in the uterus, heart, skin, testes, and small intestine.

The second system consists of CB2 receptors (cannabinoid receptor 2) that are found on immune cells. They are expressed in the immune system and other cells associated in our skin, spleen, and gastrointestinal system. CB2 cells are associated with inflammation, neuroplasticity, and forming new neural pathways.

Both CB1 and CB2 receptors act like radar. They are able to pick up biochemical signals from every organ in your entire body to help them communicate on a cellular level.

When Cannabis enters your body, the molecules interact and bind to proteins and receptors on the surface of our cells in our bodies. CBD and THC both travel through our blood stream to our brain and activates our ECS receptors. Unlike THC, CBD doesn't cause intoxication.

That's when the party starts and things start happening. While THC attaches to CB1 receptors to produce psychological effects, CBD does not activate CB1 receptors. Rather, the CBD interacts with the CB1 receptors and actually prevents THC from binding to the receptor. So, CBD reduces the effects of THC on your brain by reducing anxiety or memory issues. It helps to slow things down and keeps your brain from being over-stimulated.

Next, CBD increases anandamide. If you don't know what anandamide is, or have trouble pronouncing it, don't worry – just call it what I do – the bliss molecule! Anandamide is popular because it has a positive effect on our mood, feelings, and perceptions. It raises the levels of serotonin and dopamine in our bodies. Anandamide also attaches to our CB2 receptors and can help increase production of new nerve cells, reduce inflammation, increase creativity, stimulate the reward and motivation centers of our brains, increase memory, balance our hormones, decrease the proliferation of cancer throughout our bodies, decrease neuropathic pain, and reduce the frequency and intensity of headaches.

Recent studies have shown that CBD raises the endocannabinoid anandamides, which promote the production of macrophages. Macrophages are a type of white blood cell that your body produces that help consume cellular debris and foreign substances, including cancer cells. An increase in macrophages is related to the maintenance of intestinal balance and stability as well as increasing your immune system.

This isn't related to CBD, necessarily, but it makes me happy: if you want to keep your anandamide levels high, eat some dark chocolate!

CBD also reduces the blood flow in the areas of our brains associated with anxiety disorders. This is why CBD is helpful in reducing issues with severe anxiety such as panic attacks or post-traumatic stress disorder (PTSD.)

Another common effect of CBD is the reduction in depression. Depression occurs when there is a reduction in the pleasure components in your brain, which also includes dopamine. Activating the dopamine neurotransmitter, which CBD can do, increases the feeling of pleasure. Increasing the feeling of pleasure can alleviate the symptoms of depression. Understand, however, that CBD does not impact dopamine directly. Instead, CBD acts upon the 5-HT1A receptor which is found in many areas of the brain, especially the pleasure pathways where dopamine activity happens.

CBD has also been found to help increase attention and appetite, aid in the regulation of mood and increase happiness in general, and reduce symptoms related to cancer and the treatment of cancer.

Our brain is connected to our central nervous system. So, when we first feel pain, the sensation starts with a signal to our nerves. The nerve cells send this message to our brain cells telling the brain that we have pain. In order to find relief, the body notifies our opioid system. This is the part of our body that controls pain relief and improves our mood. After all, who can be happy when they are in pain?

There are three peptides in our opioid system: enkephalins, endorphins, and dynorphins. These peptides reduce pain. Our opioid system is commonly controlled by opiates like morphine and other narcotic painkillers. CBD has similar benefits to pain reduction, in that it acts on the opioid system in a similar way, without the harmful risks and dangerous side effects.

CBD has amazing neuroprotective effects on the CB2 receptors and is related to an anti-inflammatory response in the immune cells of the brain, therefore minimizing the amount of damage caused by inflammation.

Excitotoxicity is a process by which neural cells are killed off by over-stimulation. No, I don't mean by watching an overly exciting movie or by studying too much for school. This can happen as a side effect of seizures. It effects both CB1 and CB2 receptors. CBD can help reduce excitotoxicity by lowering the degree of excessive stimulation in the neurons, which in turn lowers the number and intensity of seizures associated with epilepsy and other seizure-related disorders. There is a new CBD drug that is being developed for children with Dravet syndrome, a severe form of epilepsy that appears in very young children. The results are so successful that as of this writing, it is now in its third stage of clinical trials!

As we age, we lose brain cells and neurons every day. Another benefit of CBD is that it influences activity in our hippocampus, which controls both short-term and long-term memory. It's also the first part of the brain which is affected in Alzheimer's patients. CBD acts on the CB1 and CB2 receptors in the hippocampus, which in turn lowers oxidation stress. It is thought that oxidation stress may be at least partially responsible for the brain damage that occurs with early stages of Alzheimer's and Parkinson's disease, and other forms of dementia.

Believe it or not, CBD can protect our brains from harm in a number of neurodegenerative diseases and increase the number of viable brain cells. Some studies have shown it to reduce the number of injured brain cells by more than 50%.

Each time you take a breath, you take energy away from your cells. Think about all of the free radical and other pollution in our air. They are adding to our system and killing off healthy cells within our bodies. They lower the number of good cells which are needed to fight off the bad cells. CBD contains antioxidant compounds which counteract oxidative stress in our cells and actually have neuroprotective effects on our brains. This creates new neurons that strengthen our hippocampus. The CB2 receptors battle oxidation in order to restore our brain function back to normal levels.

Overall, CBD is an effective treatment for a number of ailments, with many neuroprotective properties for people of all ages. Studies suggest that CBD can protect against sudden brain-damaging events, like strokes, without adverse side effects. However, as with any medical issue, you should talk to your doctor about your concerns or questions or how CBD might interact with your current conditions or medications.

BIBLIOGRAPHY

Kynaston, Herman. <u>CBD Oil for Pain Relief: A Comprehensive Beginner's Guide to Learn and Understand CBD Oil for Pain Relief</u>. CBD Oil for Pain Relief, Pub. Kindle Edition.

Lagano, Laura. <u>The CBD Oil Miracle</u>. St. Martin's Press. Kindle Edition.

Smith, MD MPH, Gregory. CBD: What You Need to Know. Kindle Edition.

Key Cannabis Terms

Bioavailability. Bioavailability refers to how much of a substance ingested or placed in or on the body is available for use in the body.

Cannabinoids. A type of chemical compound found in the human body and the body of other mammals and plants, especially Cannabis. Some subtypes of cannabinoids are CBD, CBN, and THC. A phytocannabinoid is a sub-type of cannabinoid found in a plant.

Cannabis. The common name for the plant Cannabis sativa, it is the most commonly grown variant of both agricultural hemp and marijuana (intoxicating) hemp.

CB1 and CB2 Receptors. Parts of the human immune system which are designed to receive cannabinoids. CB1 receptors can be found in the central nervous system, such as the spine and the brain. CB2 receptors are found in the peripheral nervous system, that is, the nerves that branch out from the spinal cord.

CBC. An acronym for the cannabinoid cannabichromene. It is a non-intoxicating phytocannabinoid known to retard inflammation and help the contraction of blood cells.

CBD. An acronym for the cannabinoid cannabidiol. It is a non-intoxicating phytocannabinoid found primarily in the flowers of the hemp plant, also known as Cannabis sativa.

CBD Distillates. A CBD product that, in addition to cannabidiol, contains other cannabinoids, terpenes, and plant materials. Usually, a CBD distillate product will have some THC present, and is produced from a plant that contains a higher amount of THC than a more pure CBD product.

CBD Isolate. Cannabidiol isolated from the other extracts from the Cannabis plant. All other plant matter, oils, waxes, and organic materials are removed to create a pure CBD product that is usually tasteless and in crystalline powder form.

CBG. An acronym for the cannabinoid cannabigerol. It is a non-intoxicating phytocannabinoid known to promote the growth of cells.

CBN. An acronym for the cannabinoid cannabinol. It is a non-intoxicating phytocannabinoid known for aiding in sleep.

Efficacy. A measurement to determine whether or not a product or medicine has the ability to do what it claims.

Full-Spectrum. Hemp oil made with the entire plant without isolating the CBD component. In order to be considered a non-marijuana product, it must have less than 0.3% THC. Preliminary research shows that full-spectrum products tend to be more effective than the individual components taken separately.

Hemp. Also known as agricultural hemp, this is a plant that contains less than 0.3% of the intoxicant THC.

Hemp Oil. The oil from the seeds of the hemp plant. It is cannabinoid-free, and generally used for cosmetic products due to its moisturizing properties.

Hybrid Strains. Variants of the Cannabis plant that combine qualities of both the indicia and sativa strains.

Indicia Strains. Variants of the Cannabis plant that generally grow from 3-6 feet tall, can be grown indoors, and have a sedative effect. They can also lessen pain and anxiety in some users.

Nanotechnology. In this context, nanotechnology is breaking down the product to its essential molecules so that the body needs to do the least amount of work in order to make it bioavailable. It can also mean using microscopic molecules of things like fat to coat the CBD molecules to help the body absorb the product more quickly and efficiently.

Sativa Strains. Variants of the Cannabis plant that are non-intoxicating and do not have a sedative effect. Most CBD is extracted from the sativa strains. It usually has an uplifting or energetic effect.

Terpenes. Chemicals present in the hemp plant that give the plant its characteristic odor. They also contain their own properties that aid in the relief of certain symptoms in the human body.

THCV. An acronym for the cannabinoid tetrahydrocannabiuarin. It is a non-intoxicating phytocannabinoid that helps suppress appetite and control Type II diabetes.

CBG and CBN:
Not-So-Minor Cannabinoids

CBG

CBG, or cannabigerol, is called a "minor" cannabinoid because after the plant is harvested, dried, and processed, there are only trace amounts of CBG left. That doesn't mean, however, that CBG doesn't have a major effect.

CBG is the first phytocannabinoid that develops in Cannabis, and scientists believe that it is responsible for the development of CBD and THC, and other cannabinoids as the plant matures. For that reason, it is sometimes referred to as the "stem cell" of the Cannabis plant. It's acidic form, CBGA, is the first cannabinoid acid to develop and is found in the highest concentrations in the flowering plant.

Like CBD and most other phytocannabinoids, CBG won't get you high. Early research – and isn't most Cannabis research early research? – shows that CBG can inhibit GABA neurotransmission in the brain. GABA, or gamma-aminobutyric acid, is an inhibitory neurotransmitter in the central nervous system and its job is to reduce the excitability of neurons. So, if you are reducing the transmissions and the excitability of neurons, naturally you will have less pain and inflammation. These are promising findings!

It also follows that you will experience muscle relaxation and anti-anxiety effects. Who wouldn't want that? Some of the newer studies show that it seems to have anti-depressant qualities.

The endocannabinoid receptors in the eye are especially concentrated so CBG's effect on diseases like glaucoma can work wonders.

All of these give potential hope to those who suffer from a number of conditions, such as chronic depression and anxiety, and inflammatory diseases like irritable bowel syndrome. Studies are ongoing to see how CBG affects diseases like ulcerative colitis, Crohn's disease, and Huntington's disease. Laboratory studies suggest that the anti-bacterial properties of CBG might even help prevent deadly diseases like colon cancer.

More studies are needed to determine just how helpful this "minor" phytocannabinoid can be. Some anecdotal evidence shows that it helps treat glaucoma and cancer. Of course, it is difficult to separate the effects of CBG from its cousins. CBD and THC have some of the same properties and are often present when the results are seen. But they do have different chemical makeups, so it would follow that they would have different chemical effects on the body.

CBN

CBN is a cannabinol, a mildly psychoactive phytocannabinoid. One weird thing about CBN is that as the Cannabis plant ages, its THC content breaks down into CBN.

Although CBN does have psychoactive properties, they are mild. You can get high from CBN, but you'd have to take massive doses to feel any kind of effect.

Odds are good you haven't heard of CBN until now. CBD and THC get all the press. However, CBN was one of the first phyto-cannabinoids to be identified. In the 1930s, scientists thought CBN, not THC, was the compound in marijuana that got you high, mainly because THC hadn't yet been discovered.

Despite the fact that we have known about CBN longer than we have known about THC and CBD, we know less about CBN than the others. Even so, what little we know is promising. Taken with

CBD, it seems to increase REM[2] sleep. Despite the increase in vivid dreaming with CBN, the incidence of nightmares is decreased. Sleep disorders like insomnia and sleep apnea lessen with CBN. Preliminary studies show that it works best when taken in combination with other cannabinoids, though exactly what is most effective is yet to be set in stone. Still, it is promising for those suffering from the pressure related to glaucoma and people suffering from MRSA.

The amount of CBN in a plant varies based on its exposure to heat and light. It can also change based on the age of the plant, because – remember – it's what happens to THC as it breaks down.

Because research is still in its infancy, we don't know a lot. What we do know, however, is all positive. One of the greatest things we are discovering is that CBD and the other phytocannabinoids seem to tamp down some of the negative effects of THC, like paranoia and anxiety. If we can isolate and study CBN more, it may be able to have the sedative effect of THC so people can use it for sleep without the negative side effects. Studies on mice show it increases sleep time – why wouldn't it work on us, too?

---

[2] REM stands for "Rapid Eye Movement" and this is the stage of sleep most associated with vivid dreaming.

Why We Need This Book

So many CBD stores are popping up in my neighborhood that it seems like there might be a zoning ordinance requiring a CBD store every so many feet. CBD is quickly becoming a go-to for adults, children, and even pets for just about every symptom. It is being touted for better overall health, for cancer, for sleeping problems, headaches, anxiety, pain management, and just about everything else.

That's why we need this book. We need to have a conversation about what CBD is good for, what it isn't good for, and all things in between. It is an innovative wellness product showing a lot of great hope, but it isn't a cure-all. It's hard to get good information from someone who is trying to sell you a product. I don't know about you, but I tend to not trust salespeople who have a profit motive.

A recent 2017, study published in the Journal of the American Medical Association[3] reported that less than 30% of CBD products sold in the United States were accurately labeled. Those are not good odds. So who is your trusted source to help you determine what is fact and what is fiction? It can be confusing and scary to find legitimate information about CBD products.

Unfortunately, you can't ask most doctors and pharmacists because they haven't had any formal training on medical marijuana or CBD. The majority of doctors haven't even studied the endocannabinoid system (ECS) or learned anything in medical school or residency about THC or CBD.

With the boom in the CBD market, snake oil merchants armed with misinformation and a lack of government regulation have saturated the market. You can get CBD products at a specialty

---

[3] https://jamanetwork.com/journals/jama/fullarticle/2661569

CBD store, sure, but also at spas, gas stations, and hair salons. Are these products the same quality? Do they have the amount of CBD that the label says they do? How would you know? What other ingredients are inside that bottle?

You want a product that uses a third-party, independent lab to test its ingredients to make sure that it is high quality. How do you know if this is the case? Just because the salesperson tells you it's true?

My goal in this book is to help you answer the following questions, at a minimum:

- What is CBD?
- Will CBD get me high?
- Is CBD addictive?
- How much CBD do I take?
- Is CBD good for you?
- How can I incorporate CBD into my daily wellness routine?
- Do I use CBD only when I am sick or feeling 'off'?

I have spent a long time doing research and interviewing top experts in the field. I did this to educate myself, first. Now that I know, I can educate you as a consumer of CBD. I want to help you determine the best and most appropriate CBD products for your overall wellness and happiness. This book will tell you how to make CBD work for you and how to make certain you are getting high-quality, safe CBD products.

From there, armed with this knowledge, it is my hope that you can educate your friends, elders, and peers about the incredible effects and benefits of CBD on reducing symptoms in your body caused by aging. So many of us have aging parents that let the stigma of marijuana and fear of the unknown keep them from trying CBD.

The History of Cannabis

Cannabis has been used by mankind for thousands of years. In some form or fashion, Cannabis has been used as medicine, building materials, in ceremonies, and as a textile for as long as we have known.

There are a great number of historical figures that used Cannabis. Queen Victoria used CBD-rich Cannabis to soothe her menstrual cramps. Betsy Ross, the famous flag maker, used hemp to sew her flags. Both Thomas Jefferson and George Washington grew hemp on their farms. The Declaration of Independence itself was made from hemp. While many countries historically prohibited the growth of Cannabis, England's King Henry VII fined farmers if they did not raise hemp for industrial use.

CBD, or cannabidiol, has been in existence since the end of the first Ice Age. In fact, Cannabis sativa, which is the source plant for the CBD compound, is thought to be one of the first and oldest agricultural crops planted between 10,000 and 12,000 years ago. It helped us move from being hunters and gatherers to being an agricultural society.

As early as 6,000 BCE, Cannabis oil and seeds were used for food in China. Around 4,000 BCE, the plant started to be used in China and Turkestan for textiles. By the year 1,000 BCE, rope manufacturers in Italy were using it to manufacture riggings for Italian ships.

It started being used medicinally in China, Egypt, and India around 2,600 years ago for inflammation, pain relief, anxiety, and intestinal issues. A Chinese herbalist and surgeon named Hua Tuo developed a product using Cannabis for healing and surgery at about that time.

In 1582, a Portuguese doctor named Garcia Da Orta noted its medical benefits.

Once colonization began in the western hemisphere, hemp came along with the colonizers. By 1533, Cannabis was planted by settlers in Jamestown, Virginia. Ironically, because the strong fiber was so useful, it became illegal not to grow Cannabis in the state of Virginia. Times certainly have changed.

In the 1830s, an Englishman named William Brooke O'Shaughnessy, documented the healing benefits of Cannabis. Within a few decades, doctors and pharmacies began using and selling Cannabis in the United States. By 1850, the *U.S. Pharmacopeia*, a standard reference of medicines, ingredients in foods, and dietary supplements, added Cannabis to its roles. This was a huge step in recognizing its medicinal properties, and around this time, it was commonly available in stores and pharmacies.

In 1915, synthetic drugs were introduced, and the popularity of Cannabis started to fade. This was likely due to the inconsistent quality control. The potency of extracts could vary wildly. Plant variety was a factor, and the composition of phytochemicals within each harvest changed how effective each dose was.

Once recognized by universities and medical associations as an effective medical treatment in 1942, Cannabis was removed from the *U.S. Pharmacopeia*. In 1937, the commissioner of the U.S. Treasury Department's Federal Bureau of Narcotics, Harry Anslinger, fired the opening shots in what would later become the War on Drugs. He drafted the "Marihuana Tax Act of 1937," effectively criminalizing Cannabis and hemp nationwide. What the government once required land owners to grow, the government now prohibited. Talk about a flip-flop!

The government didn't want to listen to any scientific evidence. The American Medical Association (AMA) opposed the Marihuana Tax Act of 1937 that imposed taxes on physicians and pharmacists prescribing and dispensing Cannabis and took away what they believed to be an effective treatment. Still, political pressure prevailed, and the act passed.

Unfortunately, because hemp and marijuana come from the same plant, Cannabis sativa, they were lumped together under the Act. This useful plant with its useful fiber was now illegal to grow and use. The law was designed to regulate the recreational use of marijuana and tried to do so by cutting it off at its source. It imposed heavy taxes on Cannabis growers. As a result, farmers moved away from growing hemp, and the broader association (and confusion) of all Cannabis with marijuana began.

Science will not be stopped!

The scientific research on the Cannabis sativa L plant led to the discovery of a previously-unidentified signaling system in the brain known as the endocannabinoid system (ECS.) We now know that the ECS is found in both vertebrates and invertebrates. It has diverse and significant roles in our physical and mental health. Cannabinoids are natural substances that exist within us whether or not we take them in from outside sources.

Despite this, when the War on Drugs escalated in the 20th century, the Controlled Substances Act of 1970 classified marijuana as a Schedule I drug—a designation reserved for substances thought to be addictive and have no medical applications. This effectively put a halt on research since scientists in universities and government laboratories could not legally possess marijuana to properly to research it.

It was, of course, misclassified entirely for the wrong reasons. Schedule I drugs, according to the U.S. Drug Enforcement Agency, "have a high potential for abuse and the potential to create severe psychological and/or physical dependence." This is not true of marijuana, but it gets lumped in with heroin, LSD, and MDMA anyway. Consider this: cocaine, meth, and many opioids like Oxycodone – yes, the same drugs that are fueling the opioid crisis –

are listed as Schedule II drugs. This means the U.S. Federal Government has classified them as having a *lower* potential of abuse than Cannabis. I triple-dog-dare you to tell me this was a scientific decision and not a politically-driven one.

Given the lack of good scientific research, how do we know what we know? Where there's a will, there's a way, for one. Marijuana and Cannabis derivatives never lost their mythos with natural healers. Patients who trusted the doctor-patient confidentiality and spoke of their Cannabis use were able to give anecdotal evidence about the efficacy of Cannabis in treating cancer symptoms. Word of mouth spread.

How did CBD get its start?

Extracting CBD from the Cannabis plant is not a simple task, so how did it begin? In 1940, a Harvard-trained chemist named Roger Adams was the first to extract CBD from a Cannabis sativa plant. He didn't know what to do with what he extracted but extract it he did. In 1946, Dr. Walter Loewe proved that Adams' extraction did not alter the mental state of users.

It wasn't until 1964 that Dr. Raphael Mechoulam was able to isolate and describe the chemical structure of CBD. Mechoulam also figured out that THC is the intoxicating compound in marijuana and that CBD doesn't have THC in it.

In the early to mid-1970's, the *British Pharmacopoeia* released a licensed Cannabis tincture that likely contained a full-spectrum CBD oil for therapeutic use. New Mexico became the first state in the U.S. to acknowledge Cannabis as medicine in 1978. This was known as the Controlled Substances Therapeutic Research Act. It was the first instance of Cannabis compounds legally recognized for the medicinal potential, though at the time, due to federal laws, there wasn't anything New Mexico could do other than give Cannabis a shout out.

In February 1980, Dr. Mechoulam – The Godfather of Modern Cannabis – teamed up with South American researchers to publish a study on Cannabis and epilepsy. Results of these trials revealed that subjects who received CBD experienced improvement with their symptoms, with little to no side effects. This was a monumental discovery for people with debilitating seizures.

In 1996, my home state of California became the first state in the U.S. to legalize medical marijuana. Known as the Compassionate Use Act of 1996, this legislation legalized access for people with severe or chronic illnesses. Fairfax's Marin Alliance for Medical Marijuana became the first medical marijuana dispensary to open in the U.S., and dozens of states have since followed. It is still federally illegal, but federal drug enforcement agencies turn a blind eye to medical use.

On October 7, 2003, the United States Patent Office granted U.S. Patent Number 6,630,507 that involved CBD as a neuroprotectant. This is good because it acknowledges CBD as an effective medicine. It highlights the hypocrisy of the government. However, it touts its effectiveness in one breath while insisting on keeping it on the list of Schedule I narcotics in another.

In 2009, California's Steep Hill Laboratory tested a cultivar of marijuana which is the first known CBD-rich cultivar of Cannabis in the U.S. In 2011, studies found CBD useful in treating diseases like epilepsy, anxiety, cardiovascular diseases, schizophrenia, and cancer.

The 2014 Farm Bill, including the Hemp Growers Act, made growing hemp legal again, and the floodgates opened. This bill defined industrial hemp as Cannabis sativa containing 0.3% of THC or less[4]. State agriculture departments and institutions of higher education were now able to cultivate hemp for agricultural

---

[4] By comparison, marijuana usually contains anywhere from 15% to 40% THC, the active ingredient that creates the "stoned" feeling. You'd have to smoke at least 135 times as much hemp to get as high as some weak marijuana.

purposes and academic research. Farmers interested in growing hemp could become certified by their state agriculture departments. Hemp production supervision moved from the DEA to the USDA and the FDA in 2018, opening the door to more sensible regulation. In Canada, CBD products were approved for sale under the Cannabis Act in June of 2018.

Recognizing this, more and more states are passing medical marijuana laws. In 2014, Alabama, Florida, Iowa, Kentucky, Mississippi, Missouri, North and South Carolina, Tennessee, Utah, and Wisconsin passed legislation for the legalization of medical CBD. More states are joining in all the time.

In 2015, the market saw an influx of CBD-infused foods and edibles for humans and pets. These edibles can be found in Cannabis stores in states where recreational marijuana is legal, but you can also find them in some alternative retailers in other places.

Slowly but surely, the stigma associated with Cannabis is going away and the stubborn resistance to medical marijuana by the mainstream medical community is fading. In 2017, the National Academies of Science released "The Health Effects of Cannabis and Cannabinoids: the Current State of Evidence and Recommendations for Research."[5] This group of healthcare providers and scientists reviewed tens of thousands of research, studies, and anecdotal evidence showing the effectiveness of marijuana in several conditions and noting the need for more intensive research.

Of course, money drives everything. Pharmaceutical companies don't have much profit motive to spend the millions of dollars necessary to get high quality marijuana-based pharmaceuticals approved by the FDA. The main active ingredients of any of them are going to be THC and CBD, naturally occurring chemicals that can't be patented. Without a patent, any other company could copy what they've done and take away the profit.

---

[5] https://www.ncbi.nlm.nih.gov/pubmed/28182367

In early 2020, as I am writing this, CBD supplements and products are legal in some form or fashion in all 50 states. There are exceptions, mainly depending on how the CBD was derived and from what plant, so make sure you check to avoid breaking any state laws.

Fun Facts about Cannabis and the Endocannabinoid System

It seems like no matter how much I read and research, I still have questions and I still learn something new. Here's some interesting things I found out along my journey:

- There are at least 130 cannabinoids in hemp, of which CBD is only one.
- CBD, THC, and CBG (cannabigerol) are the only three found in large quantities.
- CBD takes up 40% of a hemp plant's extract.
- CBD oil is taken from the flowers, stems, leaves, or buds, the "resin glands" of marijuana or hemp plants.
- When it was originally isolated, no one thought CBD had any pharmaceutical use.
- Conventional wisdom says that CBD taken from marijuana plants is of higher quality than CBD taken from hemp plants.
- "Full spectrum" CBD oil is usually only made with female plants.
- Everything that is alive that has a spine has an endocannabinoid system.
- The endocannabinoid system regulates homeostasis within our bodies.

The endocannabinoid system is in charge of maintaining balance and regulating:

- Mood
- Memory
- Pain perception
- Sleep
- Motor control
- Appetite
- The endocannabinoid system, like everything in our bodies, doesn't work as well as we age, and you can become "cannabinoid deficient."
- Mother's milk is rich in cannabinoids.
- Plant-based cannabinoids stimulate your natural cannabinoid system and allow your body to rebalance.
- Cannabinoid deficiencies can result in chemical-induced anxiety.
- CBD is more prevalent in the flowers and buds of the plants than the stems and stalks.
- Different strains of hemp and marijuana have different concentrations of CBD.
- Legal constraints against marijuana prevent the large-scale study of marijuana extracts.
- Cannabis sativa has two medically important subtypes: Cannabis sativa sativa, and Cannabis sativa indica.
- Sativa plants are tall and thin with long, thin leaves; indica plants are short and stout with short, wide leaves.
- The ruderalis subtype is not medically important.
- Sativa and Indica grow in the parts of the world closer to the equator.
- Sativa has high CBD and low THC; Indica has the opposite.
- Cross breeding has led to hundreds of hybrid strains with the properties of both.
- The smell, taste, color, and look of the plant and the product of the plant have nothing to do with its potency. The only way to get that information is to test it in a lab.

- Crops grown from the same strain can have different potency levels, so they each must be tested.
- CBD has a greater health impact than THC.
- All cannabinoids affect the endocannabinoid system in some way, but because of the legalities of studying them, it is hard to say exactly how.
- Olive oil and ethanol usually extract more of the terpenes from the plants than other solvents.
- Slight remnants of the solvents remain in the extract, so make sure you don't use products that were extracted with carcinogens.
- Extracts made with food grade oils like olive oil or coconut oil are great for ingesting, but they are also perishable, so they can expire.

From Seed to Soap

If you're like me, you're curious. And if you aren't curious, why are you reading this book? It's amazing to me that someone can take a seed and grow it into a plant and extract an oil from it with near-miracle qualities and then turn that into a bar of soap that can soothe my aching muscles. How does that happen?

It starts with a clone. Like we talked about earlier, each crop of plants has different qualities. Just like each child from the same parents is different, each plant from the same set of seeds is different. So, to make things uniform, the plants are cloned. This ensures that each plant has the same amount of CBD and other cannabinoids in it and has a consistent product.

Plant cloning isn't mad science. It can be done by taking a cutting from a plant and growing a new plant from the cutting rather than growing new plants from seeds. The cuttings get planted, grow, and are harvested. It takes anywhere from 108 to 120 days for a plant to be fully mature and harvestable. Once they are harvested, they are hung in a barn to air-dry. They are cured just like tobacco, hanging upside down in a dry, ventilated place to make sure they don't mildew.

Once they are dried and cured, the flower is pulled off the plants through a process called "retting." The flowers are ground down and steeped like tea in methanol to remove the compounds in the plant that give it the distinct odor we wouldn't want to walk into a business meeting smelling like. They may also be extracted using carbon dioxide, which is highly effective, but expensive. Ethanol can be used and its methods are straightforward but also potentially dangerous. Using oils to extract CBD is the oldest method – even ancient oils like olive oil can be used. Oils are safe and cheap but yield very little CBD.

However you extract the CBD, the extraction is subjected to cold. Think about when you put a fatty soup, like chicken soup, in the refrigerator – all the fat rises to the top. That's what happens here. The fatty acids and lipids rise to the top and are easily pulled off. These can potentially alter the chemical makeup of the oil, so we want to remove them.

What's left after that is distilled, and a raw oil remains. It is distilled once again to remove contaminants and to make the color clear. The terpenes, which are the active ingredients, are not removed during the distillation process.

At this point, if it's a quality product, the oil is sent to an independent lab for testing. That's the only true way to know the strength and percentages of the contents of the oil. Once the company has that information, the oil is added to other oils, and then mixed into the ingredients that make up soap, muscle balms, lotions, and even *eyebrow gel* – everything you can think of!

In a nutshell, or a bud – ha, ha – that's how you get from a Cannabis seed to a bar of soap!

PERSONAL STORIES

Dr. Paula Petry
Cannabis: The Plant Well-Traveled

It is 1968. I am 15 years old at a family gathering in northern Illinois. "I don't understand the big deal about pot. The Native Americans used to smoke it in their peace pipes," my cousin Deborah argues. Marijuana, for my aunts and uncles, was associated with long hair, mini-skirts, anti-war protests, and flag burning; they all looked aghast. No one seems to be convinced, I thought to myself. In fact, no one left the family reunion persuaded, other than Deborah, that marijuana was a good thing. I left tempted to try it and curious as to whether Native Americans actually did smoke marijuana in their ceremonial pipes.

Decades later, as a shamanic energy medicine practitioner, I find the historical geography of Cannabis and how it was frequently intertwined with spiritual, religious, and medicinal practices interesting and important to Cannabis' emerging importance in modern medicine. Its multitudinous uses and benefits help explain why this plant, over so many others, is so well-traveled – having traversed millions of miles and five continents to have reached the Americas in the 19th century.

This chapter begins with a brief description of Cannabis, its taxonomy and medicinal qualities. It will then explore ways in which the plant has had a consistent presence in religious, shamanistic, and medicinal applications across Asia and Africa.

What is Cannabis?

One of the most common classifications of Cannabis was created by Carl Linnaeus in 1753, i.e. *Cannabis sativa* and *Cannabis sativa L.* The Cannabis genus *sativa*—along with its sleepier relative Cannabis *indica*—is a hardy, rapidly growing plant that averages up to twenty feet in maturity. Its psychoactive chemistry is attributable to a sticky resin that the female plant produces that is rich with cannabinoids. The most important of these cannabinoids is delta-9-tetrahydrocannabinol (THC), identified by two Israeli biochemists in 1964. The THC induces psychological and sensory effects such as an altered sense of space and time, euphoria, a sense of oneness, a heightened sense of creativity, and increased introspection (Zablocki et al.,1991). This subspecies has been an extensive part of religious ceremonies and rituals across the world. It has been known by many monikers, including ma in China; Sanskrit khanap, Arabic kif; bhang, charas, and ganja in India; and dagga in parts of Africa.

Cannabis *sativa L.* has no psychoactive chemistry and is also referred to as hemp in the literature. It is equally hardy and fast growing as her sister plant. It is rich in cannabidiol (CBD), an all-natural, non-psychoactive compound found in the Cannabis plant. It grows in warmer climates and its leaves are narrower and it flowers longer than the *sativa*.

It is important to note that the taxonomic history of Cannabis is complicated. The translations often use the terms Cannabis and fiber-rich hemp interchangeably, leaving uncertain precisely when psychoactive Cannabis was used. Also unknown is the degree to which the plant described had non-psychoactive cannabinoids such as cannabidiol (CBD), which may have been present in varying degrees in ancient fiber biotypes as well as drug biotypes (Brand et al., 2017). Therefore, when and whether we can overlay today's taxonomy onto historical uses of Cannabis remains opaque.

Beginnings

Cannabis evolved as early as 12,000 years ago. Though the exact source area is in question, much of the research suggests that. Cannabis *sativa's* origin was on the steppes of temperate Central Asia in Mongolia and Southern Siberia. While Cannabis *sativa L* originated in the Hindu Kush mountains in South East Asia. (Clark et al., 2013). They are among the oldest cultivated plants on the planet. The archaeobotanical evidence of its spread focuses on pollen and seed analysis; however, ancient documents and other artifacts provide a more complete picture of its cultivation and use.

Central Asia

As early as 3000 BCE, Cannabis seeds were associated with funerary ceremonies. In Central Asia, the seeds were found in a Kurgan burial mound along with grave vessels, weapons, and horses (Godwin, 1967). Similarly, large quantities of mummified psychoactive Cannabis were found in the tombs of nobles buried in Xinjiang, an autonomous region in the far northwest of modern-day China and Siberia, around 2500 BC (Russo, 2004).

China

Cannabis *sativa L* has been cultivated in China for millennia for use as fiber, food, and medicine. References to Cannabis are found in many famous works of philosophy, poetry, medicine, and agriculture (Brand et al., 2017). The medicinal uses of Cannabis were first documented in the *Divine Farmer's Classic of Herbalism* (Shen Nong Ben Cao Jing), compiled 2000 years ago and attributed to the works of Shen-Nong, China's legendary Fire Emperor who lived 4500 years ago (Ferrara, 2016). Shen-Nong is said to have investigated the properties of several hundred herbs, the beginnings of what became Traditional Chinese Medicine. In this holistic approach to well-being, excess psychological factors known as the "seven emotions" are thought to affect disease development. Each of these emotions—joy, anger, sadness, anxiety, worry, fear, and fright—interact with particular internal organs, leading to patterns of disharmony. In the document's descriptions for Cannabis, the resinous female inflorescence of the Cannabis plant is said to be effective in treating the seven emotions listed above. Cannabis was also thought to help with exhaustion, a weak pulse, problems with one's organs; it was also used as an anesthetic in surgeries (Merlin, 1972).

Contemporary research into pre-modern Chinese medical texts, known as bencao, explored the historical uses of different parts of the Cannabis plant. The study's primary reference was the authentic editions of over 800 historical bencao texts (Brand et.al., 2017). Special attention was given to reviewing the application of Cannabis for seizures, pain, and mental illness. The plant parts associated with concentrated cannabinoids, female flowering tops and leaves, were emphasized. Surprisingly, there were only a small number of compound formulas that featured the use of *mafen*, the female inflorescence, albeit its effectiveness, as seen in the example above. Another entry, by the physician Sun Simiao (581-683 AD), describes his use of the extracted juice from crushed Cannabis leaves to treat unbearable pain due to fractured bones. Similarly, one entry describes soaking its seeds in water, which is thought to have yielded cannabinoids. Exposing broken resin glands to heat would have recreated bioavailable THC. This compound relieved "pain from the inability to move." In the seventh century, Cannabis was listed as an effective treatment for wind-withdrawal, a set of symptoms analogous to today's use of the term mental illness (Brand et al., 2017).

Shamanism, the oldest of spiritual traditions, creates a seamless blending of ritual, ceremony, mythology, healing, and divination. The identification, knowledge, and use of plants were central to their role, as physician, psychologist, and priest. Their use of

Cannabis and other psychoactive plants to access higher wisdom is well documented; there are over 275 psychoactive plants used by shamans globally (Tedlock, 2005). Shamanic knowledge and applications of medicinal plants was passed forward as societies evolved. These practices in China were prominent up until the Han dynasty (206 BCE–220 CE) when it was suppressed. At that time shamanism merged with an early form of Daoism as a way to keep the practices alive (Ferrara, 2014). Although references to Cannabis in Daoist literature are relatively infrequent, there are several notable inclusions. Cannabis was one of the many ingredients in the herbal and mineral drinks used to aid the process of inner exploration. Highlighted in *Essentials of the Matchless Books* (Wu Shang Pi Yao), a sixth-century anthology, is the practice of burning Cannabis to drive away evil ghosts.

Also, the Daoist encyclopedia *Wushang Biyao* (Supreme Secret Essentials) records Cannabis used in censers (Needham, 2014). Cannabis and other herbal medicines used in conjunction with a censer was associated with fire, combustion, dissolution, communication with spiritual beings, and assurances of immortality. This represented change and the spiritual transformation Daoists were seeking. It was part of the religious Daoist's quest for the "Elixir of Life" and gaining transcendence over human mortality (Ferrara, 2014).

Another indication of the veneration of Cannabis is Ma Gu - the Hemp Maiden (Abel 1980). A beautiful young woman described as having long, birdlike fingernails and carrying a green plant, Ma Gu is seen as the protector of females in Chinese mythology. Historian and sinologist Joseph Needham described Ma Gu as the goddess of Shandong, an eastern coastal province of China, sacred Mount Tai, where Cannabis "was supposed to be gathered on the seventh day of the seventh month, a day of seance Taoist banquets," (Needham, 2014).

Korea and Japan

By 2000 BCE, hemp and Cannabis found their way to Korea and Japan. It is believed the nomadic herds of Mongolia and the Middle East were responsible. Rope imprinted pottery, seeds, and woven fibers dating back to the Jomon culture (10,000 BCE - 300 BCE) supports its early presence (Clarke et al., 2013). In Shintoism, the largest religion in Japan, the priests waved bundles of burning hemp to cleanse the shrine of potential evil spirits. Hemp was associated with purity and brides wore veils made from hemp on their wedding day. Although with the rise of Confucianism during the Han Dynasty (206 BCE - 220 BCE), the ingestion of the psychoactive Cannabis was suppressed in China; its use in Japan is not clear.

India

Cannabis arrived in South Asia between 2000 and 1000 BCE, through the established trade routes. In high contrast to China, Mark Ferrara describes India quiet differently, "marijuana-growing and its consumption probably reached its greatest efflorescence" (Ferrara, 2016). To that point, Cannabis is identified as one of the five essential plants in the Vedas, Hindu religious texts. Bhang is made from the leaves and flowers of the female plant, which results in a high level of cannabinoids, which according to the Vedas, have healing properties. A guardian angel is described as living in its leaves and providing joy and happiness. She was seen as a liberator to help humans be released from fear (Abel, 1980). Its medicinal uses were expansive, including rabies, epilepsy, and anxiety.

Bhang is widely mentioned throughout the *Rig Veda* (Bennett, 2010), one of the world's oldest religious texts, dating from 1700–1100 BCE. It is a collection of Vedic Sanskrit writings that refer to sacrifices, rituals, and praises for various gods. It is one of the four Hindu religious Vedic texts, and the basis of a system of health care known today as Ayurvedic medicine. The *Rig Veda* contains more than 1,000 hymns organized by mandalas; many are verses and melodies venerating the gods, while others are for various sacrificial rituals. The *Atharva Veda*, or "Science of Charms" refers to bhang as one of the five most sacred plants (Bennet et al., 1995). In one section, bhang is identified as a protector and preserver of life. It reads,

"With the herb that brings delight,
Amulet given by the Gods,

We in the conflict overcome illness and all
Rākshasas [demonic beings].

May Cannabis and Jangida [herbs] preserve
me from Vishkandha [illness],

—that Brought to us from the forest, this
sprung from the saps of husbandry.

(Ferrara, 2014).

Another well-known Hindu text is the *Bhagavad-Gita*, interpreted to mean "the Song of God" or the "Divine Song". Through a story that takes place on a battlefield, Arujuna seeks counsel from Lord Krishna as to what would be considered right action; going into battle meant killing his cousins, uncles, fathers, and their sons, potentially bringing bad karma to him and his family. The teachings awaken Arujuna's esoteric understanding of karmic law. He does go into battle, living true to his warrior caste, but does so unattached to the outcome. In this story, Bhang is mentioned as a way to sharpen the memory and alleviate fatigue (White, 1971). In fact, all throughout ancient India, bhang was known to improve the intellect, cure dysentery, aid digestion, and give gaiety to the mind and alertness to the body.

The serious religious intention associated with Cannabis is reflected in the veneration of the Hindu God Shiva, referred to fondly as the "Lord of Bhang." During Shivaratri, a holy festival to honor Shiva, bhang is consumed in his praise and to give thanks; bhang, Shiva's favorite food, is a mixture of crushed psychoactive Cannabis leaves mixed with nuts, spices and sugar, and then boiled in milk. Ganja, another term for Cannabis, is burned and exhaled in abundant offerings to Shiva. These celebrations were a way to induce peak-experiences, higher states of consciousness, sense of oneness, and unity with God.

In India, Cannabis sativa is a plant that was unquestionably thought to contribute to one's physical, mental, emotional, and spiritual well-being. The gods were depicted drinking it, the religious texts explained ways to use it, and a special drink made with bhang, spices, and milk was part of ordinary life. The reaction of the British colonialists to this extensive use of a psychoactive plant should not be surprising. In the late 1800's the House of Commons of the United Kingdom commissioned a large-scale study throughout India for the primary purpose to address their concern that the use of bhang and ganja was leading to psychosis (Iverson, 2008).

A thousand standardized interviews later, including 1200 doctors, visits to asylums, and years of detailed analysis, the appointed Indian Hemp Drugs Commission Report produced its six volumes of data and conclusions, a total of 3,281 pages. The Commission did not find any reason to suppress the use of Cannabis sativa. They concluded that in moderation, Cannabis is harmless to physical, mental, and emotional health. In addition, they stated that prohibition could possibly lead to the use of more dangerous narcotics.

Egypt

It was the Scythians who brought Cannabis into Egypt, sometime between 2000 and 1400 BC (Warf, 2014). The Scythians were nomads who lived in an area once known as Scythia, an area in modern day Iran and areas of Eastern Europe. Their use of Cannabis is well documented in both funerary rituals and for mind, body, soul purification. The purification rites took place inside small tents where Cannabis seeds were heated on stones. As the fumes rose up, they were inhaled, followed by a "howling with joy" chanting experience (Warf, 2014, 422).

Once in Egypt, its medicinal properties were recognized and incorporated into Egypt's evolving knowledge of herbal medicine, as witnessed by *The Ebers Papyrus*, the oldest and most important ancient record of herbal medicine in Egypt, dating around 1500 BCE, but based on older records from around 2640 BCE. The papyri used a hieratic script similar to hieroglyphics in what is a 110-page scroll, containing 700 formulas and folk remedies. It is organized by chapters with categories that we would find in a modern-day medical textbook, i.e. intestinal disease, ophthalmology, dermatology, gynecology and obstetrics, dentistry, and surgical treatments. *The Ebers Papyrus* recommended Cannabis remedies were for such ailments as uterine contractions, inflammation, sore toenails, fever, and gonorrhea.

Goddess Seshat is the Egyptian goddess of wisdom, knowledge, writing, and astrology. She is found at many sacred sites, including Karnack, in Luxor. She is thought to have invented writing and helped measure and transcribe the dimensions that were to be used in the construction of temples and pyramids. Her glyph is a long stem with a seven-pointed leaf and a crescent moon shape above the leaf, sometimes with a small opening mid-way.

The leaf's shape has an uncanny similarity to that of Cannabis. In researching the leaf's significance, the explanations seem incomplete. In communication with a colleague and tour guide for trips into Egypt, Trista Haggerty reflected, "Perhaps the seven points represent the seven planets so revered by the Egyptians, and the arch above could represent the soul 'housing' the planets." That seemed to have possibilities in the context of another hieroglyphic text that reads, "Seshat opens the door of heaven for you," (Ferrara, 2014) which suggests that Seshat was perceived as a bridge between worlds, thus her link to astrology and her star covered body. As we have seen in other cultures, the morphology of Cannabis makes possible communication with the cosmos. Cannabis pollen was found on the mummy of Ramses II who died in 1213 BCE. The Cannabis may have helped transport him to the world beyond death.

All told, Cannabis existed or was diffused into every major geographic region in the world. It was entwined in the world economy and was part of religious, social, and medical practices and part of everyday life. It has been venerated, marginalized, and demonized as its landscapes changed. Today with the aid of modern science, the thousands of years of ancient chronicled medical records have turned into complex laboratory analyses of its chemical compounds and controlled studies of its healing properties.

This is creating, what appears to some, a new narrative but recorded history tells a different story. Cannabis as a legitimate and beneficial health substance, is of course not novel. In fact, this reemergence of Cannabis represents the cyclical nature of time and how time flows back onto itself; the future reaches back to pull us forward, a classic example of an ouroboros, the image of a snake or dragon eating its own tail.

Northern Illinois 21st Century

Perhaps my cousin's 1968 quip, "I don't understand the big deal about pot," should have been, "Pot is a big deal." Not only for the Native Americans who in the 1900's incorporated it into their already existing sacred pipe ceremonies, but for the multitudes who came before and after. In August 2013, Democratic Gov. Pat Quinn signed the Compassionate Use of Medical Cannabis Pilot Program Act. Its opening paragraph reads,

(a) The recorded use of Cannabis as a medicine goes back nearly 5,000 years. Modern medical research has confirmed the beneficial uses of Cannabis in treating or alleviating the pain, nausea, and other symptoms associated with a variety of debilitating medical conditions, including cancer, multiple sclerosis, and HIV/AIDS, as found by the National Academy of Sciences' Institute of Medicine in March 1999.

On January 1, 2020, the use and sale of recreational marijuana went into effect in Illinois. It joins eleven other states in legalizing recreational marijuana and thirty-two other states and the District of Columbia in legalizing medical marijuana.

If the Cannabis plant could talk, it may say:

"For logic to prevail, it sometimes takes longer than anyone could ever imagine. I am grateful to continue my service. Now, let me again help you preserve your good health; live with less pain and more joy; find a calm inner state; stimulate your appetite; and lift the veil between worlds so you can access higher wisdom."

References

Abel, E. (1980). *Marihuana: The First Twelve Thousand Years.* New York: Plenum Press.

Bennett, C. (2010). *Cannabis and the Soma Solution.* Waterville, OR: Trine Day.

Brand, J. E., Zhao, Z. (2017). Cannabis in Chinese Medicine: Are Some Traditional Indications Referenced in Ancient Literature Related to Cannabinoids? *Frontiers in Pharmacology.* Volume 8 article 108.

Clarke, R., and Merlin, M. (2013). *Cannabis: Evolution and Ethnobotany.* Berkeley: University of California Press, 2013.

Ferrara, Mark S. (2016). *Sacred Bliss.* Rowman & Littlefield Publishers. Kindle Edition.

Godwin, H. (1967). The Ancient Cultivation of Hemp, *Antiquity* 41:42-9.

Hillig, K. W., and Mahlberg, P. G. (2004). A chemotaxonomic analysis of cannabinoid variation in Cannabis (Cannabaceae). *Am. J. Bot.* 91, 966-975. Doi: 10.3732/ajb.91.6.966

Iverson, L. (2000). *The Science of Marijuana.* New York: Oxford University Press.

Li, H.-L. (1974). An Archaeological and Historical Account of Cannabis in China. *Economic Botany* 28 (4): 437-448.

Merlin, M. (1972). *Man and Marijuana.* Teaneck, N.J.: Farleigh Dickinson University Press.

Needham, Joseph (1974). Volume 5, Chemistry and Chemical technology; Part 2, *Spagrical Discovery and Invention: Magisteries of Gold and Immortality. Science and Civilisation in China.* Cambridge University Press.

Pierce, David (Not Available) *Chronic Spirituality: The History of Cannabis.* Books 4 A Better Life. Kindle Edition.

Russo, E. (2004). History of Cannabis as a Medicine. In *Medicinal Uses of Cannabis and Cannabinoids,* edited by G. Guy, B. Whittle and P. Robson, 1-16. London: Pharmaceutical Press.

Schlosser, E. (2004). *Making Peace with Pot.* New York Times 26 April, p. A23.

Tedlock, B. (2005). *The Woman in the Shaman's Body: Reclaiming the Feminine in Religion and Medicine.* New York: Bantam Books.

Warf, B. (2014). High Points: An Historical Geography of Cannabis. *Geographical Review* 104 (4): 414-438.

White, D. (1971). Human Perfection in the Bhagavadgītā. *Philosophy East and West,* 21(1), 43-53.

Zablocki, B., Aidala, A., Hansell, S., and White, H. (1991). Marijuana Use, Introspectiveness, and Mental Health. *Journal of Health and Social Behavior* 32 (1): 65-79.

About Dr. Paula Petry

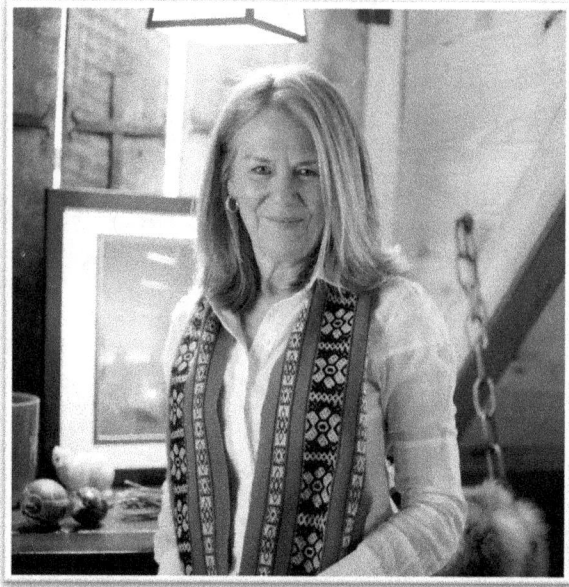

Dr. Paula Petry is an author, speaker, presenter, and shamanic energy medicine practitioner. She is passionate about helping other women awaken to their inner world to find peace, self-worth, passion, and purpose.

Her memoir, *A Mother's Courage to Awaken: Finding Hope and Inspiration with my Daughter in the Afterlife* explores death and resurrection, broken dreams, and a life transformed beyond whatever was imagined possible. It is a story about the love for and loss of a precious child and the healing quest that loss initiated. Paula resides part-time in Miami, Florida and Cooperstown, New York where she is a co-owner of the Light of Heart Sanctuary.

www.PaulaPetry.com

Avianna Castro

Tell me about your journey with Cannabis and your area of expertise.

I became aware of CBD during a discussion with friends about the upcoming legalization of the product. Cannabis is typically considered something with a negative stigma that should be avoided. I have never smoked, not even a cigarette, or used any recreational drugs in this lifetime. There has never been a pull or desire to do so, not even to this day.

My purpose in this lifetime is connecting to Spirit and I do this through being an intuitive and meditation teacher. Having anything disrupt that connection does not allow for a desired outcome. So, when I was offered CBD, I had my reservations because I associated Cannabis with getting high. I was unaware of its benefits. Through research of CBD and THC, I began to realize the effects of CBD mimic a compound already found within us and can harmonize and align homeostasis in the body. Once I became more educated, I began to understand and trust in the research being done with CBD. This along with the beneficial effects I had heard through testimonies, I was open to trying CBD.

Being a meditation teacher, my personal practice and what I teach is to go within. So many of us have immense stress, whether it be with our career, family, relationships, or our own health. I believe part of our challenge in society is to reach for something tangible to "fix it." Meaning, we have become an addictive society choosing to look to the outside to find peace instead of going within. Going within requires space, time, patience, letting go of what we think we know, as well as listening to and building our spiritual "muscle". Our world has become filled with chemicals being over prescribed and not even coming close to solving the problem. I believe CBD is a natural conduit to assist many people and animals, helping to heal the body without the negative side effects or addictions to chemicals. I truly believe there is a time and place for medicine. However, I don't believe it is necessarily the first thing we need to reach for to improve the health of our bodies, minds, and souls.

When did your interest in Cannabis start and why?

In 2017, I became more educated in the medicinal properties of CBD. I used it on occasion, but it was not something consistent in my daily practice until mid 2018. It was at that time that my beloved therapy dog, Gracie, started limping. After taking her to the vet, we learned she had a cranial cruciate ligament (CCL) tear which is similar to an anterior cruciate ligament (ACL) tear in humans. There is no treatment for this type of injury other than surgery. The worst news though, is that once a dog has a CCL tear in one knee, it is very common for the other knee to endure the same injury. While waiting for surgery, we monitored her closely but you could tell she was uncomfortable. It was during this time that someone reminded me that CBD is also available for pets and I should consider using it to help with her ligaments and pain. As parents, whether to human children or our animal children, we would do anything to ease their discomfort naturally. Trying CBD oil for Gracie felt to be a safe and beneficial option. Literally, within hours of giving her CBD, her limping minimized and she was feeling better.

Over the course of the next several months, we continued giving CBD to Gracie. We headed into surgery in April 2019, to repair her right knee. Her surgeon knew and supported the use of CBD because he saw the progression of her healing. I gave Gracie her CBD the day before surgery and continued it immediately following surgery.

At our two-week checkup, the surgeon asked what she was on and I told him CBD. He was amazed with her healing and progress made in such a short amount of time after surgery.

CBD is being utilized more and more in alternative ways of healing. As soon as we got home from her initial surgery, her left knee began to fail. We knew what we were up against, but we also knew we were better equipped for her recovery.

Post-surgery on both knees, Gracie is back to running and climbing stairs. It is truly magical watching her be able to be a dog again. What I saw in her completely changed my awareness of the beneficial effects of CBD even for my own personal use.

Give me an example of how Cannabis was life changing for someone you know.

I have heard countless stories of how this amazing healing plant can help improve lives. From seizure disorders to chronic diseases going into remission, to aiding the body's natural ability to restore itself to a healthy state. I have seen it with our Gracie as well as with several others. I also believe that people who want an alternate way to heal will also need to let go of the negative connotation of the plant medicine as I had to. As with anything, I feel intention of use is essential. Our intentions were to heal and assist, going to the core of the issue.

How has Cannabis helped you, clients, and others where other products were unsuccessful?

In July of 2019, I was introduced to a new nanotechnology delivery system being used with CBD. I felt a difference within hours of trying this new formulation. When we have experienced the benefits of this product, our own personal story becomes more credible. For me, the Nano CBD was a game changer. Along with owning a thriving meditation studio, providing intuitive and mediumship consultations, speaking engagements, hosting retreats, as well as several other projects, my schedule is very hectic. While I have a lot on my plate, I don't experience anxiety, but I do experience the energy of being overwhelmed. This newer Nano-technology CBD balanced this energy allowing me to avoid becoming overwhelmed, to be more focused, and able to efficiently accomplish more throughout the day.

I want to emphasize that this new product has a profound yet subtle effect. I am very sensitive and even certain "natural" ways to increase energy create a heart racing effect. This product did not have that effect on me and it was amazing how clear things became. I knew that I wanted to invest in the product and add it to our line of services at the studio. We purchased our first order and sold out within days! The product has provided amazing results for everyone who has tried it. People are more focused, getting deeper sleep, have relief from pain, have more joint flexibility, and even an increase in feeling more confident. I must add though, at the studio we provide a holistic approach. We teach about using products in addition to a deep meditation practice, connecting with nature, journaling, as well as a gratitude practice. I truly believe in healing on all levels that align with the soul, our infinite wisdom, and without that, our healing may indeed not be as profound.

What changes in the industry do you foresee coming in the future?

I feel the Cannabis industry will continue to thrive. Without proper education and awareness, I believe there will be many who will not consider this route to health and healing because of the stigma that surrounds Cannabis as a whole. I do know several people, including medical professionals, who are not in support of this medicinal product. But there are also many others who do. Often, people will accept advice from someone because they have a title, not necessarily because the advice provides the best outcome. To help avoid this in my own personal life, I interview my physicians so that the alignment of health and wellness is in harmony. Unfortunately, we live in a world that is fueled by money, but it is my intention to help shift it to be a world fueled for the health and wellness for everyone without a price attached to it. As this industry continues to flourish, it will be important for people to do their own research and become more educated on what products/lines are good for them.

Like anything else, there are quality products and ones that fall short. I encourage people to sample and feel the energy of the products to make sure there is an affinity. For me, I knew instantly when there was an alignment of a product that worked for me; my body immediately felt the difference. For example, I am one who dreams but has a hard time remembering them. I have never had trouble falling asleep, but while using the product, I got a deep, restful sleep full of dreams that I now remember. I sleep fewer hours a night, but I feel more rested upon waking. While taking the product, I found it fascinating that it helped me sleep soundly at night and then in the morning, it helped me get energized and focused. It seems a bit counterintuitive, but I believe this is the intention of the plant. It has an intuition of its own knowing and aligning to what the body needs in order to be harmonized. Plant medicine with conscious properties connecting to the oneness of our earth with all its inhabitants who choose to take it with pure intention is powerful!

I believe this is exactly why I was finally open to receiving the message of this medicine. A natural medicine from the earth that coalesces with the energy already within. Simply, let that be what heals us. Technology is absolutely amazing, but sometimes going back to our roots in the most natural and organic way is the best way to heal. I feel we are moving in this direction and in time, the re-evolution of this plant will be what provides healing to many lives.

The programs of the human mind can be incredibly rigid and confining. It is unfortunate that many can experience profound ways of healing only if open to go beyond the traditional ways of doing things. I am so appreciative of trusting in those who gifted it to me and that it was available to support in the healing of our Gracie. I invite everyone to be open to trying CBD in order to experience its subtle healing properties. Honor the process of organically healing from the root. Over time, the healing can take place at a level that is not felt. Honor it, trust it, and welcome it as a facet of wellness.

About Avianna Castro

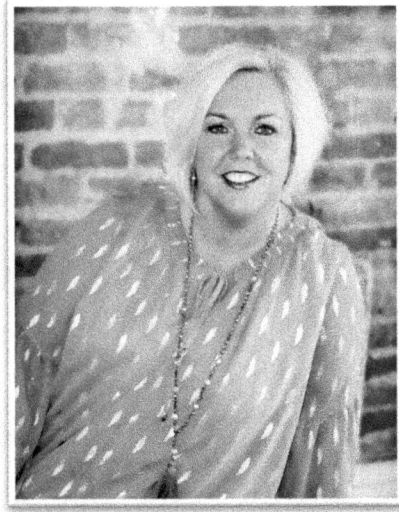

Avianna Castro is an entrepreneur, intuitive medium, awareness mentor, and meditation teacher. She is a Certified Meditation and Mindfulness Teacher with the McLean Meditation Academy in Sedona, Arizona, as well as a Chopra Center Certified Instructor in Primordial Sound Meditation. She is also currently a member of the online faculty at SWIHA (Southwest Institute of Healing Arts) teaching mindfulness and guided imagery courses.

Avianna has also received her Past Life regression certification through Dr. Brian Weiss at the Omega Institute and is actively offering regressions and progressions for her clients.

Avianna's most passionate endeavor has been the opening of her meditation studio in Flushing, MI. Bringing consciousness to the community is her dharma and now she has a beautiful studio to share her love of life. She is passionate about helping others cultivate inspirational change through intuition, awareness, mindfulness, and meditation. Avianna empowers others to live awake and authentic, creating a reality that is spiritual and meaningful.

Avianna works with adults, children, businesses, physicians, colleges, and universities such as the University of Michigan and Michigan State University to encompass mindful awareness and meditation into daily life integrating presence, clarity, guidance, and peace.

Brian Essenter

Tell me about your journey with Cannabis and share your area of expertise.

My career in Cannabis started rather like many other things in life. I was in the right place at the right time and knew the right people. It was not something that was at all planned.

In 2012, when Connecticut approved its Medical Marijuana Program, it mirrored the regulations of retail pharmacies and required pharmacists to run the medical marijuana dispensaries. At the time, I was aware of this development but, like many other people, I was very skeptical that the program would even survive. I discussed that possibility with my wife and we decided that the risk might not be worth it just yet.

The Medical Marijuana program went live in September 2014. A few months earlier, the Connecticut Pharmacists Association sponsored a four-hour Medical Marijuana Symposium Continuing Education program. It was here that I learned a good friend and colleague was going to be leaving the same retailer we both worked for to open one of the first six medical marijuana dispensaries in the state. We had an in-depth conversation about the industry, and I mentioned that if he were aware of any openings to let me know because I was interested.

A few months later, while on vacation, I got a call from a dispensary owner who was looking to replace her current Dispensary Manager and was given my name and contact information. I am still not sure why I answered the call because it was an unknown number and I was on vacation. I guess it was divine intervention.

Everything happened so fast that my wife and I were just trying to make sure things stayed mostly the same with such major changes that seemed out of nowhere. We were still apprehensive because we had a very young daughter. We did not want the opinions of other families to cause any issues for our daughter so we didn't tell anyone about my new job for the first 6-12 months. The last thing I wanted was for someone to not let their child be friends with my daughter because of some outdated stigmas.

To our surprise, most of the people I did tell were extremely supportive and many were curious. They were very happy for me to be involved in an industry that is experiencing such rapid growth. Because it was a new and topical industry that few knew much about, most asked a lot of questions. Others told me stories about friends and family members that were currently using or were interested in using Cannabis to help treat their symptoms. Overall, our friends have been very supportive which I believe is because I am a pharmacist and I consider Cannabis a medication that should be treated with respect. If it is dosed and used properly, it can alleviate many symptoms that patients experience daily without having to smoke or get high. When I speak about Cannabis, most realize that we are taking a very scientific approach to helping our patients medicate appropriately and safely.

The ability to help patients directly improve their quality of life and become more active participants gives me goosebumps every day! Most pharmacists go to school to graduate and help people. In retail pharmacy, it is extremely difficulty to help patients directly and have an impact on their healthcare. Most of your time is spent fighting with the insurance companies and doctors about what is covered, what isn't, and why. At the same time, corporate offices give you more responsibility but take help away from you. These conditions made it very difficult to have any conversations with patients about their prescriptions or healthcare in general.

In the dispensary, it is the complete opposite experience. We have direct patient contact on a regular basis. We have the time to talk to the patients and discuss how to adjust their current therapy in order to achieve better symptom relief with fewer side effects. And in the process, we are also able to help patients adjust their prescription medications safely!

For me, the best part is when the patients come in to the dispensary crying (happily), laughing, hugging, and high-fiving because they are using a walker instead of a wheel chair, or a cane instead of a walker. Many share stories of getting off prescription medication or having their cancer markers decreased (or sometimes even complete remission). Other are happy just because they were able to play on the floor with their grandkids or simply enjoy a meal with loved ones! These are the reasons we wake up every morning and go into work with a smile on our faces.

We have some of the strongest and most determined patients! They have been left behind by "conventional medication." Doctors have not been able to solve the issues with pills, so they just give the patients what they ask for because they don't have the time or take the time to try something different. Patients want to have some control over their own healthcare. They do not want to feel like a lab rat when their insurance company tells their doctor the new medication he prescribed is not covered and they try a cheaper medication which fails.

At the dispensary, the patient makes the final decision! This is a huge part of what makes the medical marijuana program so successful! The patient gets to choose which delivery method, which strain, when, and how to medicate. They can medicate to the level needed. Most people are not experiencing the same amount of pain, depression, anxiety, seizures, nausea, or difficulty sleeping EVERYDAY! So, it is only natural to be able to adjust your medication to your needs. Also, giving patients the ability to adjust their delivery method allows them to control the onset and duration of the effect for their specific need.

We must remember that every patient is different. If two patients have the same cause of their pain, it does not mean they will only benefit from using the exact same strains. Every patient has compounding factors that can lead us to suggest a different path of medicating. These factors could include whether they are working or not, have kids, or have additional conditions (cancer, Parkinson's, MS, epilepsy) that might not be visible at that moment. These are more reasons why it is so important for a healthcare professional to be able to help! And, I am proud to be one of them that is doing so!

When did your interest start in Cannabis and why?

My interest in Cannabis started in college as it does for many. I found a medication that I felt was great at helping me deal with the stresses of college, difficulty sleeping, and social anxiety that many in their teens and early twenties encounter. I found that I (and MANY others like me) were using this plant to medicate rather than using prescription medications.

After college, I worked in pharmacies and had to stop using Cannabis for a few years. I found that life had become more stressful; I was not sleeping well (or at all sometimes), and the prescription medications I was given to help were causing side effects that affected my work during the day. So, the prescription medications ended up making things more complicated instead of helping. It wasn't until I found Cannabis again that I was able to get a good night's sleep and handle my stress levels in a much more responsible and productive way. I also noticed that Cannabis was helping me with my aches and pains.

After moving to Connecticut and working in retail pharmacy for 16 years, I was given an opportunity to manage a medical marijuana dispensary. In Connecticut, pharmacists were required to work in dispensaries so they could also counsel patients on their prescription medications. Also, pharmacists already knew how to work within regulations set up by the state regarding controlled substances. This opened an unusual door for me as a pharmacist who had seen firsthand how Cannabis could help where prescription medications have not.

Once I started working in the dispensary, I found out very quickly that I was not nearly as knowledgeable as I believed I was. Pharmacists often have big egos, and I am no different. In my first couple of days at the dispensary, I realized that my patients knew more about these products that I did. And, I was the one who was supposed to be making the recommendations. I made it my mission to learn everything I could about the delivery methods, strains, and what we had available.

I found that it was not difficult to find good information as long as you look in the right places. And, the more information I found, the more information I wanted to find! It is unbelievable how much information there really is out there if you just look.

As a pharmacist who had taken many science classes, it was a little easier for me to be able to decipher the good information from the "questionable." But the information I thought was true yesterday might be completely different tomorrow. The science and research being done in the Cannabis industry is mostly outside of the United States because of our archaic federal laws.

So as a pharmacist, you also need to be willing to adjust your opinion and information that we discuss with our patients. That may be the most difficult thing about this industry – the science is changing so quickly that in order to stay current, you really do need to be doing research every day! And, it is still possible to be outdated which is another reason why I love this industry.

The biggest takeaway is that no matter how much anything changes in this industry, in the thousands of years Cannabis has been around, it has still never killed anyone! It has the safest profile of any medication that currently exists and can benefit in ways we haven't been able to figure out yet!

What are the misconceptions of Cannabis?

- You do not have to smoke or get high to achieve symptom relief
- Cannabis is not a gateway drug
- Cannabis is safer than alcohol
- Cannabis has less than a 9% addiction rate

What questions are you most frequently asked?

1. How do I find the best CBD product?
2. Do I have to smoke?
3. Do I have to get high?
4. Can I stop my prescription medications?
5. Can I travel with marijuana now that it is my medication?

What questions should patients be asking?

- Do you have a list of the ingredients in the preparation?
- Do you have third-party testing available?
- Can I get high from this product?

What is the recommended dose of this product? Give me a few examples of a positive experience, benefits, or success stories.

I have so many success stories that it seems like too many to tell. Very few of our patients after trying Cannabis feel that that it is not for them. The vast majority of people who try Cannabis (at least medically) continue to use it in some fashion.

However, I have helped two cancer patients achieve and so far, maintain complete remission from their cancer after their doctors said no more treatment options were available for them.

The majority of success stories I've witnessed involved patients looking to decrease or eliminate their prescription medications.

Most specifically, their opiate medications. We have helped patients with the highest dosage opiate prescriptions decrease their doses significantly, and even completely. Many of these changes were forced on patients when Connecticut changed its prescribing laws limiting the number of opiate tablets that could be prescribed to a patient. This left patients in a tailspin, looking for something that was not heroin!

Many patients had already used Cannabis at some point in their life, and now they are happy to embrace it again. Especially if it means they can feel better and not make the same bad choices many others have during our current opiate crisis. I am not saying that Cannabis can or will stop our opiate crisis, but it sure can give these patients a much softer landing. And, these patients are some of the most vulnerable people in our society.

I have also seen patients who suffer multiple seizures each day that remain uncontrolled while on prescription medications, but once on a regimen of CBD and THC, they are able to control and significantly limit the frequency and severity of the seizures. We allow them to resume a significantly more normal life.

What is the recommended starting doses for a client? Can you overdose? Are there any side effects?

Starting dosage is based on a person's history with Cannabis, their tolerance level, and their desired delivery method. The delivery will determine the time of the onset of the effects and the duration of these effects. Depending on one's tolerance to Cannabis, the side effects will vary. Side effects include feeling lightheaded, dizzy, groggy, giggly, or hungry are more typically what is referred to as being "high." We try to avoid these by accounting for a patient's ability to tolerate the side effects of Cannabis. To date, there have been no documented overdoses of Cannabis! From the latest data I have found, the dose necessary to overdose on Cannabis would require a patient to inhale 1500 pounds in under 15 seconds. And, in this case, one is more likely to die from asphyxiation than anything else.

The main concern with Cannabis is using too much THC which leads to paranoia and panic attacks. This is usually more likely to happen with edibles because of the longer time until onset and the longest duration (approximately eight hours) of any delivery method. For this reason, we try to be more aware of the individual's tolerance and very slowly titrate to the effective dose while attempting to keep side effects ("the high") to a minimum.

Dosing may also need to include more CBD than THC to make sure that the patient remains clear headed and functional. CBD can offset the lightheaded, dizzy, and drowsy effects of THC; therefore, having significantly higher CBD levels than THC (5:1 or 10:1 CBD:THC ratios). However, every patient can still be affected by the THC regardless of the levels of CBD, depending on their sensitivity to THC.

How has Cannabis helped you, clients, or others where other products were unsuccessful?

SLEEP! Pain relief! Anxiety without the drowsiness or grogginess!

What changes in the industry do you foresee coming?

- More consistent product availability
- More consistent strengths
- Better standards for manufacturing and processing
- Federal regulation

What do you wish people knew or understood about Cannabis?

It's not the "Devil's Lettuce" that everyone wants to believe it is, and it's not your parent's Cannabis either. Cannabis now is much more potent than it was 20-30 years ago.

Cannabis is a flowering plant that produces "cannabinoids" that have not been available to people in their diet or otherwise available for decades. When hemp was being used for textiles, it was also being used as feed for livestock. These animals would then have cannabinoids in their system, so we were getting cannabinoids naturally through our diet when we would consume these animal products. When Cannabis was moved to a Schedule 1 status, it was no longer part of our natural diet.

Humans have an Endocannabinoid system that consists of CB1 and CB2 receptors. These receptors are only activated by Cannabinoids. Cannabinoids do not act on other receptors such as mu receptors like opiates. Therefore, tolerance to other medications/drugs does not correlate with tolerance to Cannabis. Every patient is different no matter how similar their conditions or symptoms are. That is why there are so many different varieties of Cannabis. We each need to find the right strains that work best for us. This can be a longer process than people might normally be comfortable with. However, it is better than going to the doctor every 30 days to change anti-depressants, pain medications, anxiety medications, sleep medications, or even blood pressure medications. Patients can change their strain, dose, and delivery method at their own speed and comfort level. This allows patients to take control of their healthcare!

What is important to look for when selecting a Cannabis product?

First, look for or ask about third-party testing. Was it tested for molds, mildews, pesticides, and heavy metals?

Then, ask what delivery methods are available.

You have had such a powerful and resilient life. What message would you like to give cancer patients about Cannabis usage?

You do not need to smoke it or get high! Regardless of how bad you think things are now, they will probably get worse. Prescription medications can only do so much, and they come with significant side effects. Cannabis can be used palliatively for cancer patients to help with pain, nausea, appetite, sleep, anxiety, and even depression. Depending on your willingness to try, there are cancer protocols out there that have been shown to be effective.

I have helped two cancer patients go into complete remission after being told by their oncologists that no other options were available. Now, this is not a true scientific study. Had I not seen it with my own two eyes, I would not necessarily believe it. Recently, scientists in Spain were able to show that high doses of both THC and CBD cause tumors to slow their growth and cancer cells to go through apoptosis (spontaneous cell death). There is much more research that needs to be done before we can have any true scientific conversations about this level of treatment. But I do believe it is possible if the patient is willing and able to try.

What can we do today to start educating the public about Cannabis?

I believe that education needs to start with medical providers –doctors, APRN's, pharmacists, and nurses. Schools need to at least start talking about it and should be educating its students on the Endocannabinoid System (ECS). The ECS regulates most of the homeostasis (balance) of our bodies. It is imperative students in medical fields learn how the ECS interacts with our CNS, Immune system, Cardiac system, and our Pulmonary system.

Then, there is a need for public education to drop the stigmas and the obviously biased and racially-charged federal regulations around Cannabis. The public includes our legislators. Just because they have years of stigma behind their fears does not mean that there are not true medical benefits to Cannabis. Cannabis is safer than alcohol and tobacco, which have little to no medical benefit.

How can we make sure we provide the public with a guideline on buying the best products and the bad stuff out there?

The best advice I can give to anyone looking to purchase Cannabis products (over-the-counter CBD products or medical marijuana products) is that you make sure the seller has documentation of third-party lab testing. This is especially important for the unregulated CBD market. Most states have testing standards (some much more stringent than others) that the producers and retailers must abide by. But, the bottom line to purchasing the best products for you is to do your research before making a purchase online or walking into a store. Ask questions. You are your own best advocate (tell them what YOU want)!

Brian Essenter, RPh

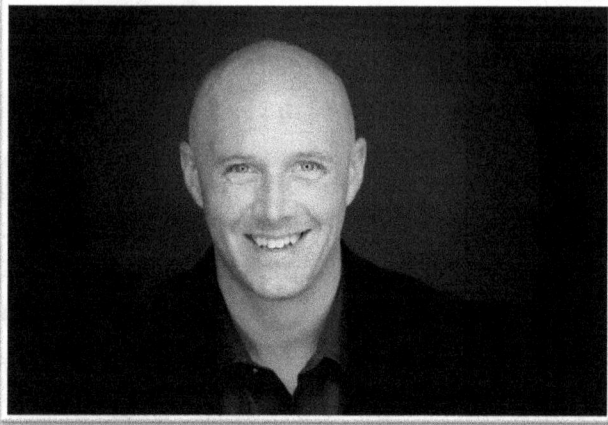

Brian Essenter, RPh is a graduate of Northeastern University and a registered pharmacist. Brian worked for one of the nation's largest national retail pharmacy chains in MA, NV, and CT for 16 years. Brian was also a dispensary manager at one of the busiest dispensaries in Connecticut for almost three years.

Brian is the owner of MM Consult CT. At MM Consult CT, Brian's goal is to answer any and all questions regarding the benefits of medical marijuana. He is also able to guide patients through the difficult process of navigating Connecticut's Medical Marijuana program. This can include suggested dosing and delivery methods appropriate for the patient's condition, as well as desired results.

Brian has consulted for businesses in the Cannabis industry and those interested in entering the industry. He has also had the opportunity to speak to many different audiences regarding medical Cannabis. Most recently, Brian consulted in opening and currently manages Affinity Health and Wellness, a medical marijuana dispensary in New Haven, CT.

Bunny Egerton

The times, they **aren't** a changin'.

January, 1972. Walker Hall dormitory. Any college, USA. I am poised in the bathroom, hand hovering over the toilet. The alert has sounded; the police are on campus, going from dorm to dorm conducting a drug raid. My sweaty hand clutches a "nickel bag," ready to flush. All the toilet stalls are similarly occupied.

The drug "scene" was, if not escalating, certainly gaining notoriety on campuses across the country. Amphetamines, pot, hash, Quaaludes, LSD; I was 18 years old and completely naïve. On the night I graduated from high school in 1971, I drank two whiskey sours - the first time I imbibed alcohol. Why didn't I drink at high school keggers? Because I knew my dad would kill me!

While I was aware of classmates smoking pot, well, see above sentence about my father!

I arrived on campus; my father was four hours away; everyone was drinking and smoking and I embraced the, "when in Rome" philosophy. But, only as far as pot was concerned. The others scared me so I stayed away.

Getting caught with pot was still a scary proposition. I knew that this would result in expulsion, jail time, family shunning, and a lifetime of misery, so the trick was not to get caught!

Choose suppliers wisely. Be discreet. And, at the first hint of troopers on campus, be certain to commandeer a stall!

I never was caught, and I enjoyed getting high.

Fast forward. I am no longer in college and no longer smoking pot. Pot was still in wide use and was easily purchased in the suburbs where I resided. I knew it was there, but I was no longer interested.

Until my brother in law was diagnosed with cancer. Forty years had passed, and it was now 2001. Surgery, radiation, chemo, hair loss, skin burns, and nausea. Modern drugs to curb side effects were not approved yet. It was a known fact that marijuana could lessen some of the side effects – particularly, it could lessen nausea and increase appetite (remember "the munchies").

It was also a known fact that pot was still illegal - and still available.

Christmas, 2001. My brother-in-law is in the hospital in Washington, D.C., for a week-long chemo regimen, and his doctor is out of town for the holidays. His mother-in-law, aka my mother, Joanie, is visiting me for what feels like a year but is actually 10 days.

We determined that a Christmas Day trip to the hospital was in order. The hospital in Washington, D.C. The hospital with a security desk to clear (we are post 9/11). Are you beginning to see where this is going?

I handed a package to MIL/Mom/Joanie – a brown paper bag tied with a big red bow.

"What is it?"

"Christmas present for your son-in-law."

"But what is it?"

"A surprise – and you are lousy at keeping secrets, so you will have to wait until he opens it. Just keep it safe until you give it to him."

The 45-minute drive from Columbia, MD to Washington, D.C. was uneventful and somewhat comical. MIL/Mom/ Joanie kept that gaily-wrapped paper bag on her lap and proudly marched it past security at the hospital.

My brother-in-law and sister were playing Scrabble when we arrived, and MIL/Mom/Joanie proudly handed over the package. She barely gave my brother-in-law time to open it before her, "What is it? What is it?", and when he showed her the contents, she still asked, "What is it?"

It was a bag of pot, and MIL/Mom/Joanie, at the age of 73, was a mule! Something I reminded her of until the day she died!

But how silly that we had to resort to this subterfuge to bring comfort to my brother-in-law. For pot. (For those of you who are wondering, after a lot of chemo, a lot of surgery, and I presume, a lot of pot, my Brother-in-Law is healed and is alive and well as you read this. And, I presume, still smoking pot!)

2018 brings another shift – medical marijuana is now an option, and clinics are opening at rapid rates. In addition, CBD has now become a "thing," and entrepreneurs are promoting this trend. Oils, gummies, cookies, all designed to ease pain, anxiety, and sleep woes without the psychoactive effect of THC, are becoming available (for the record, CBD was first discovered in 1940, but has recently enjoyed rising popularity).

And again, use is on the sly with dispensaries taking multiple precautions to avoid any legal entanglements. Perhaps we can understand the reticence to promote pot because it is a mind and mood-altering psychoactive drug. But, Cannabis *without* the THC?

Back to 2018. A good friend was suffering from two diseases which caused pain, sleeplessness, and irritability. In other words, a compromised standard of living. The solution – a girls' trip to Las Vegas, where one of the three of us had a connection to a gentleman who has been one of the pioneers in opening dispensaries to provide CBD products.

The experience put me in mind of hovering over the toilet or using an old lady as a mule…56 years after that college experience! We were buzzed in and had to show our IDs before we were taken into a small consultation room away from any other customers. There, we were shown the menu, and we indicated desired items on a sheet of paper and everything was paid for in cash that was sent through a chute so none of the employees ever actually concluded a sale.

The compromised friend was a skeptic but gamely bought about $300 worth of product. AND, became a convert. She could sleep. Her pain was eased. She enjoyed golf again. There were no side effects, ill effects, or mental changes. She wanted to refill the lotions and creams, and replenish the edibles. Hopefully, without the need to travel to Las Vegas again.

It seems that after 56 years, we should be further along than this. It seems that if we can provide relief to people without affecting their cerebral function, we should embrace this opportunity and run with it.

It seems that this book is the vehicle to dispel the myths, celebrate the successes, and open the way for Cannabis to takes its rightful place in the world.

CHARLOTTE "BUNNY" EGERTON

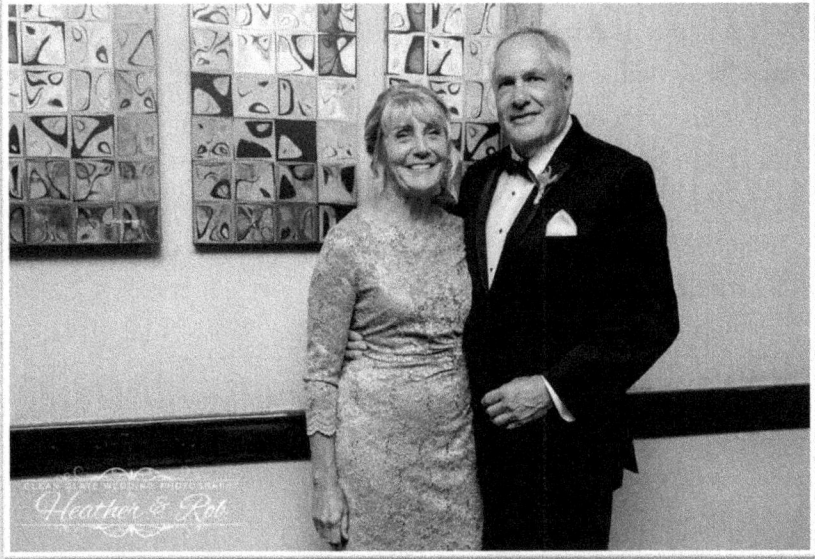

CHARLOTTE "BUNNY" EGERTON has a B.A. in English Literature and a B.A. in Secondary Education; she earned a Master's Degree (M.Ed.) in Special Education, and a Master's Equivalent in Human Resource Management. She is certificated as a Secondary English Teacher and as an adult instructor in Special Education in the state of Maryland and is licensed as a Trainer by the Maryland State Department of Education.

Currently, Charlotte is a Partner in Raising Munchkin, LLC, a training and consulting firm. She has presented teacher training and adult leadership workshops at educational and leadership conferences across the country.

Previously, Charlotte served as the General Manager for Youth Services at Columbia Association, a community non-profit organization focused on enhancing the quality of life for the residents of Columbia, MD. She also worked as the Director of Education at Foundation High School for at-risk teens located outside the District of Columbia and was an Adjunct professor at Howard Community College in the English and Education departments.

Charlotte is a perennial traveler, having climbed Mount Fuji, the Great Wall of China and Machu Picchu, hiked to the bottom of the Grand Canyon, sailed the Galapagos, camped in Nigeria, and rode along on a safari in Namibia. She has also traveled extensively throughout 50 states, Europe, Iceland, and Asia. Travel allows her to discover her greater self and share these experiences with friends and workshop participants.

Carli Jo Cabrera

Tell me about your journey and story with Cannabis. What is your area of expertise?

Although I've been a consumer of Cannabis since high school, it wasn't until recently that I started pairing sex with Cannabis with intention. As a student of Tantra in a yearlong program, I was spending hours learning, discovering, and playing with my own sexuality. I struggled A LOT with being present during sex with my partner, as well as myself. My brain wouldn't shut off; sometimes it would be negative, projecting things that weren't true. Other times, I would go to random thoughts that really didn't need to be there. Most of the time, the underlying emotion was shame.

I spent a year with the intention of being present with my body. One day, after spending a weekend meeting local Cannabis farmers from NORCAL, I was sitting in my Sacred Sensual Space doing a Tantric breathwork ritual when I got the idea to pair Cannabis and tantra. Prior to this, Cannabis was solely used recreationally. The idea of bringing it INTO the bedroom had not occurred to me. I created a beautiful ritual, smoked Cannabis, and had the most amazing sexual experience to date!

From there, my love affair with Mary Jane evolved.

When did your interest in Cannabis start and why?

My love affair with Cannabis began when I was 13 years old living on my parent's farm. My older brother was way cooler than me and I looked up to him and wanted him to think I was cool, too. He consumed Cannabis, so therefore I did as well. My mother, always sweet and sometimes naive, found a baggie of weed in my brother's jeans when doing laundry.

She eyed it, shrugged, and placed it on the dryer. I acted cool, waiting until she left, then grabbed the bag and hid it in my childhood safe. Several weeks later, my brother was throwing a party. He said, "Man, I wish I had some weed."

This was my chance!

"I have some." I said, oh so casually.

Although I smoked that night and many nights after, it wasn't until several years later that I experienced my first "high."

What are the misconceptions of Cannabis?

1. Cannabis is a gateway drug.
2. Cannabis makes you lazy.

What questions are you frequently asked about your topic?

1. What strain of Cannabis is best for sex?
2. So, like, you just get high and have sex?
3. What exactly does a Cannabis Sensuality Coach do?
4. Does Cannabis increase libido?
5. Does Cannabis intensify orgasms?

What questions should people be asking?

1. How can I introduce Cannabis into my sex life?
2. How can Cannabis ease menstruation/menopause symptoms?
3. How can I create a ritual with Cannabis?
4. How can I create a sex-positive home?

Give me a few examples of a positive experience, benefits, or success stories.

One couple in particular was having a really hard time being playful with one another. Sex had become something of a chore that would often lead to frustration. I suggested a light edible that they would each take at the beginning of the session. I asked that they share when they started to feel a difference.

About 30 minutes later, in the middle of a touch exercise, they both started giggling uncontrollably. After several minutes, the wife said, "I think it kicked in." I left them to continue the intimate practice on their own to which they messaged me later saying, "We didn't have sex, but OMG we needed that carefree, fun, and playful experience!"

One client who paired Cannabis and tantra said, "I felt feelings I've never felt in my body before. Feeling sexual urges as if I am f*cking like a King."

What is the recommended starting dose for clients? Can you overdose, and what are the side effects?

When it comes to pairing Cannabis and sexy time, you don't want to overdo it. Getting too high can cause you to pass out or experience paranoia. The best practice is going low and slow.

Start with low doses of Cannabis, then wait and see how you feel before consuming more. Keep in mind that no two experiences are the same; Cannabis will impact you differently every time.

How was Cannabis life changing for someone you know?

Many men (more than you think) suffer from erectile difficulties. I was working with a couple who'd been struggling with mismatched libidos. The woman, feeling frustrated and rejected, the man, feeling inadequate and incapable of pleasing his woman, came to me for help. He was considering taking Viagra when I offered a more natural solution. Sour Diesel, nature's Viagra as they call it, has been known to work wonders on men's erectile function, performance anxiety, and confidence. It worked so well that they joked that when she was ready for sex, she'd pack him a bowl!

How has Cannabis helped you, clients, or others where other products were unsuccessful?

Cannabis has worked wonders for women who struggle with the side effects of our monthly bleed. For years, I tried over-the-counter meds such as Midol, which left me feeling disoriented and disconnected from my body. Cannabis-infused suppositories have been the most successful and natural product for easing pain and stress.

What do you wish people knew or understood about Cannabis?

My wish is for every soul to educate themselves on the emotional, physical, and spiritual benefits of Cannabis. Pairing Cannabis and sex has many benefits such as increased connection, libido, and desire while decreasing performance anxiety, sexual shame, and erectile difficulties. In fact, there are many potential sexual benefits to using CBD, but one of the most notable is the cannabinoid's potential to help with erectile dysfunction. This is largely due to its ability to repair tissue damage and improve blood flow to the genitals. CBD has the ability to naturally boost one's energy and is a stress reliever.

About Carli Jo Cabrera

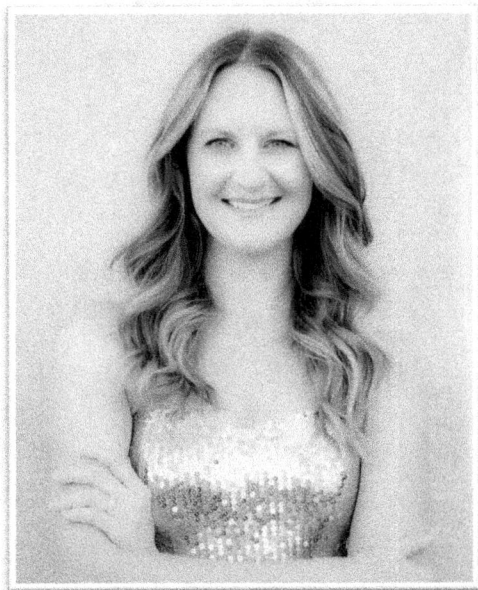

Carli Jo is an educator on becoming your own Sexpert, Sex, Love & Relationship coach and Cannabis advocate who helps couples become lovers, women become orgasmic, and all souls achieve greater sexual satisfaction.

Author of *Your Itty Bitty Guide to Cannabis and Sex,* Carli Jo uses sacred sex practices with plant medicine to weave together ancient healing and spiritual methods that are playful and effective.

Janet Macksood

Tell me about your journey with Cannabis and your area of expertise.

My journey in the world of Cannabis began approximately five years ago when my father was diagnosed with Parkinson's and Dementia. The pharmaceutical medications he was taking were not helping control many of his symptoms (shaky hands, not speaking full sentences, paranoia, and outbursts). When he reached a plateau from the medication, I had to find an alternative to treat his symptoms and give him the quality of life he deserved. I researched plant-based medicine, which led me to Cannabis.

I began giving him concomitant therapy including 10 mg of CBD and 10 mg of THC. After the initial dose, he was speaking in full sentences, eating more, the tremors in his hands lessened, and he was comfortable. I knew we were onto something amazing that other patients could benefit from as well. As his disease progressed and he suffered multiple strokes, I began formulating different dosages and using other product forms. After a year on 10 mg of THC and straight CBD oil, he began to plateau. I continued my research into different companies and other plant- based medicines. That's when I came across Mike Williams, the creator of 5280 Nano Technologies. After comparing several other brands, I found Mike had the most progressive patent-pending Nano CBD on the market. The benefits of Nano CBD vs. oil is increased absorption and quicker onset.

I found the best dosage for my father was 20 mg of THC given during the day and 10 mg of Nano CBD liquid at night to help him sleep. After my father lost his battle in late May of 2019, my mother, who was suffering from osteoarthritis, was diagnosed with leukemia. We continued to see the benefits of the Nano CBD and how it helped relieve her pain and anxiety. I experienced the benefits of Nano CBD and the difference it made in my parents' lives.

Through my personal experience, I realized there was an extreme need for a Nano CBD consumer product line to help individuals who are suffering as my parents did. My business partner, Kristi Rohr, and I started working very closely with Mike Williams to better understand the research proving Nano CBD is much more effective than CBD oil. The benefits of Nano CBD vs. oil CBD are astounding! Kristi and I immediately founded NanoCore CBD with the goal of creating the BEST Nano CBD products for the public. Our product line consists of liquids, pain creams, edible chocolates, green drinks as well as CBD treats for dogs with joint pain and anxiety. We are passionate and committed to continuously finding ways to offer Nano CBD to the marketplace.

When did your interest start in Cannabis and why?

I spent most of my career as a medical sales representative in both pharmaceutical sales and cardiac medical devices. I had a nice understanding of how the body functions at a cellular level, the bioavailability of medications, as well as their side effects. When my father became ill, I was determined to find an alternative therapy and give him the quality of life he deserved.

What are the misconceptions of Cannabis?

One extremely common misconception is that the CBD from Cannabis will get you high. I find much of society lacks education and cannot differentiate the effects of THC vs. CBD.

Another educational weakness is that most people are only familiar with THC and CBD. Cannabis contains over 500 compounds—cannabinoids, terpenoids, omega fatty acids, and flavonoids. All of these compounds play a significant role in the benefits of Cannabis. There are over 100+ cannabinoids identified in the plant, but only a few have been fully researched. THC, CBD, CBG, THCV, CBN are the most common. Cannabis has fewer side effects and is more effective in treating ailments than most synthetic chemical-based medications.

A third misconception I've found is that all consumer CBD products are the same. CBD isolate is the most common form as well as the cheapest on the market. Unfortunately, CBD isolate is less effective in potency and absorption than Nano CBD.

What questions are you most frequently asked?

1. What is Nano CBD?
2. What is the difference between Nano CBD and CBD oil?
3. Can you get high from taking CBD?
4. Will CBD show up on a drug test for my work?
5. Is it safe for my pet to take CBD?

What questions should people be asking?

1. Are your CBD products Nano CBD or oil CBD?
2. Has the oil been tested?
3. Can I see a copy of the lab results?

What is the recommended starting and titration dosing? Are there side effects or concerns when using Cannabis?

When starting any new medication or herbal supplement, start with a low dose to ensure there are no allergic reactions and then gradually increase, if needed. Nano CBD is much more potent than regular CBD oil. Nano CBD has been broken down to an extremely small particle size, which is easier and faster for the body to absorb.

I recommend following the dosing guidelines listed on the products you purchase and always speaking with your physician when starting any supplement.

Give me a few examples of a positive experience, benefits, or success stories.

The first success story was my father (read the story above).

My personal experience with Cannabis was after I had a full hysterectomy. I did not want to take the pain medications prescribed by my doctor. I tried 10 mg of THC for pain for several days following surgery and then took 10 mg of CBD to help me sleep and reduce night sweats from the hormonal changes in my body. This has helped my sleep patterns and my mood, and I am able to get the rest needed to wake up refreshed the next morning to start my day.

One of the most heartfelt stories is from one of our customers who was diagnosed with Glioblastoma. He was having difficulty getting out of bed, having seizures, and experienced daily pain. He started taking our Nano CBD and within a few days, his seizures were less frequent and he was able to get up pain free. His quality of life and time with his family has improved immensely.

Another customer of ours had her torn meniscus cleaned out and was still in a tremendous amount of pain post-surgery. She previously tried an oil-based CBD product on the market and had minimal pain relief. She then tried our Nano CBD and had a significant decrease in pain and increase in mobility. She is now back doing the activities she was prior to her meniscus tear.

We've also had numerous pets that have greatly benefited from our NanoCore CBD Pet Treats. My own dog, Macksy, was starting to slow down at the age of 10. I began giving her a few of our CBD treats daily. Macksy became more energetic, playful, and was able to go on long walks again.

These success stories with our Nano CBD happen every day, which is why I will continue creating the most effective, innovative CBD products on the market, for others to benefit from.

Give me an example of how this was life changing for someone you know.

I have witnessed several friends who have had success taking Nano CBD for multiple reasons including headaches, anxiety, hormonal hot flashes, night sweats, aches and pains, arthritis, seizures, and muscle soreness after working out or running.

I have a close friend who has neuropathy in her hands and feet and uses our Nano CBD orally and in a lotion to relieve her pain. It has been life changing for her to be able to relieve some of the pain and inflammation she experiences on a daily basis. She can now drive her kids to school and feel confident in her ability to have motor function in her hands and feet.

I also have several family members and friends who are runners. Due to the strong anti-inflammatory properties in CBD, their recovery time is lessened, and they find relief to sore muscles after a long work out.

Another life-changing example I've witnessed is a friend of mine who suffers from anxiety when flying. So much so, that she would avoid family trips. She now takes 20 mg of Nano CBD before getting on a plane and she's able to travel for business and pleasure.

How has Cannabis helped you, clients, or others where other products were unsuccessful?

I have seen Cannabis be very effective in people who had been taking long-term prescription medications. With the use of CBD, they have been able to cut back on these strong pharmaceuticals.

In terms of CBD, I see it every day where our Nano, water-soluble products are much more effective than the current oil based products on the market. There is no comparison!

What changes in the industry do you foresee coming in the future?

I foresee education increasing and the public becoming more aware and knowledgeable about CBD products. Consumers will soon have the information they need to differentiate between the good products and the bad. Consumers becoming more savvy will increase demand for premium products, forcing companies to become more advanced in the types of seeds they plant, the quality of the soil used, as well as moving towards a cleaner way of extraction.

There will also be more research done on Cannabis showing additional benefits, resulting in more innovative product offerings.

What do you wish people knew or understood about Cannabis?

I wish people would take the time to truly understand how Cannabis works in the body and the differences between THC and CBD. Cannabis is not just a drug that allows you to get high. It has more medicinal properties than most plants and is more digestible and easier for the body to metabolize with fewer side effects than the synthetic pharmaceutical drugs forced on patients today. Also, it's important to know that the plant is 100% usable and recyclable. After the buds and leaves are extracted, the stalks and roots are used to make many more products. There is no waste and it will not overflow our landfills.

I also hope that consumers become more educated on CBD and realize that the majority of the market today is overflowing with subpar products made with oil. Consumers need to ensure that the CBD products they purchase are made with Nano CBD.

How can you tell if one Nano product is better than another?

Whether it is THC or CBD, I believe in the science behind nanotechnology. It has a more potent formula, faster onset, and higher bioavailability. The biggest difference is in the particle size of the product. A simple water test will show you if the product is good or not.

Place a few drops of product in water and if it dissipates and turns clear, then it has been processed properly and has a very low particle size. If it has a milky consistency and/or doesn't dissipate to a clear liquid when added to water, then the CBD isn't high-quality and your body will not metabolize it as fast.

I feel that all consumers need to be educated on a product and its ingredients. Just because it has a fancy label or it's on the store shelf doesn't mean that it is a good quality product. This is exactly why I created the product line NanoCore CBD – I wanted to develop a brand of high-quality products that consumers can trust.

About Janet Macksood

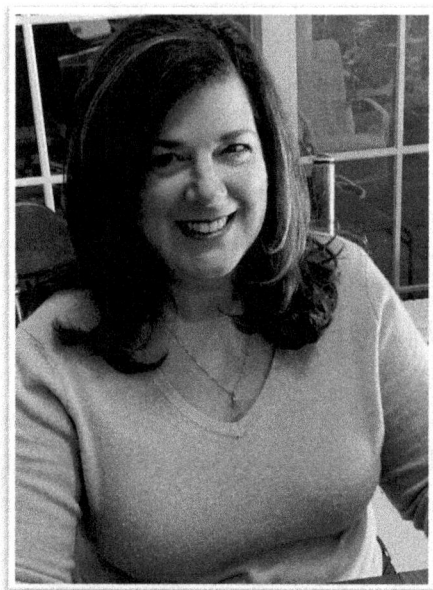

Janet Macksood is a leader in the world of sales and business development. After graduating from Oakland University with a Bachelor of Science and HR Management, Janet began her sales career with Schering-Plough and Meda Pharmaceuticals. Janet's success helped her make the transition from pharmaceutical sales to surgical sales with Sorin USA, where she aided cardiac surgeons in the placement of cardiac rhythm devices. Janet's hard work resulted in her achieving the top sales rank and winning the prestigious President's Club award.

Janet then founded Asteria Management Company where she helped numerous companies with corporate culture, infrastructure, writing business plans and running operations, sales and marketing departments. Through Asteria, Janet was introduced to the Cannabis world. During this time, her father was diagnosed with Parkinson's and Dementia. It became Janet's goal to find the best CBD available to help him. Not only did she find the most advanced Nano CBD and help her father, she also founded and launched NanoCore CBD and NancoCore Pets. These companies offer the most effective CBD products for both humans and our four legged friends. Janet is extremely passionate about the healing aspect of CBD and will continue finding innovative ways to bring additional products to market.

Dr. Michelle Ross

Tell me about your journey with Cannabis.

I grew up in a strict family, and marijuana was not part of my life. In fact, we lived across the street from a crack house, and my goal was to become a scientist who could end drug addiction. I never in a million years thought I would become one of the leading voices in Cannabis medicine and drug policy reform.

Marijuana is a drug that can affect your performance in school, make you smell bad, cause brain damage, and might even give you schizophrenia. My slacker first boyfriend smoked marijuana to drive his parents mad. I avoided it at all costs in high school and only had my first hit off a joint in college after drinking and being goaded by a boy I liked. I felt dizzy, confused, and scared of what I might do under the influence. I vowed never to smoke weed ever again.

Fast forward to graduate school where, in the Molecular Psychiatry department, I was working on a study for the National Institute on Drug Abuse to show the effects that "drugs of abuse" had on the brain. Drugs of abuse included nicotine (found in cigarettes), THC (or the scientific term Cannabis – found in marijuana), and MDMA (found in ecstasy, cocaine, methamphetamine, and heroin). I didn't use Cannabis, mostly because I worked with drugs delivered directly from NIDA like cocaine and heroin, and a positive THC test would kill my career. Also, I lived in Dallas, Texas, and very few people had Cannabis.

Doing research for my very first paper on Cannabis (and synthetic cannabinoids) to determine whether these could actually grow or kill brain cells, we found that cannabinoids can grow brain cells. I was supposed to be studying all the "bad drugs" or drugs of abuse and instead found that some of these psychedelic drugs, including Cannabis, were actually good for the brain. I ended up studying heroin and cocaine instead because they harmed the brain, but the wheels in my head were turning. I read everything I could about this mysterious endocannabinoid system and Cannabis.

When did your interest in Cannabis start and why?

After earning my PhD in Neuroscience in 2008, I moved to California from Dallas, Texas. This was the first time I had been in a state where Cannabis was legal (for medical marijuana at the time) and people were openly using it. I got to see how the industry worked and meet patients. I was pulled to take what I knew from my research and apply that knowledge to helping patients and working within the industry.

In 2013, when I founded my nonprofit—which was originally called The Endocannabinoid Deficiency Foundation (ECDF)— there wasn't a lot of research in this space in the United States. There also wasn't a lot of education about using Cannabis for women's health or Lyme's disease or autoimmune disorders - all these niche disorders.

We know so much more about them now – but at that time, we understood CBD for seizures or Cannabis for patients with terminal cancer or HIV. But, no one quite understood how to use Cannabis, or even minor cannabinoids, for other conditions. That sparked a fire in me. I'm a scientist; I'm always learning. So, when I heard that Cannabis has the potential to treat so many conditions, but no one really knew how to explain it or really how to practice it – I got really excited.

One morning in December 2011, I woke up and my right hand and wrist were completely limp and in pain. This lasted for two months. A doctor informed me that my right ulnar and radial nerves weren't sending messages through my arm. I needed an expensive surgery that might not work or could even cause permanent paralysis in my arm. After two months of trying every alternative healthcare trick in the book, it was a combination of Cannabis and hours-long massages of a "cold spot" in my arm that released the inflammation and slowly got my nerves to wake up.

I now know that I have chronic inflammation and neuropathy, and that I need daily constant consumption of Cannabis, in all its forms, in order to have functioning nerves in my arms and legs. After an initial learning curve, I discovered how to be a Cannabis patient and not only a functioning scientist and patient advocate, but a leading one.

I experienced more health issues (hello, black mold and lead poisoning from a home I rented) and I ended up a pulmonary embolism survivor with fibromyalgia. I was taking prescription drugs on the advice of my doctor (and as a downside of being on Medicaid) and they were horrible. I weaned myself off of them with Cannabis and now I only use Cannabis for my treatment.

When you consume Cannabis yourself and you realize it is the solution to your health problems, it makes you passionate for not only treating patients but for educating them as well. As a neuroscientist with fibromyalgia, I knew it was my calling to help other women with fibromyalgia get off pharmaceutical drugs and finally heal with Cannabis, kratom, mushrooms, and mindset work. I created my *Freedom From Fibro* online 12-week program to create a #FearlessFibroSquad around the world (www.Cannabisforfibromyalgia.com).

What is your area of expertise?

I've worked in many areas of Cannabis, from apps to books to product and business development to PR to patient advocacy to clinical research to lobbying to nonprofits. I'm a serial entrepreneur at heart, and that's one of the reasons why, even with a PhD in Neuroscience, I decided to get my Executive MBA, which I earned in May 2018.

I've published several books inside and outside of the Cannabis space, including *Vitamin Weed: A 4-Step Guide to Prevent and Reverse Endocannabinoid Deficiency* in March, 2018, and I'm currently working on *Gateway to Hope: CBD For Mental Health.*

I've created several online courses for my own company and other companies. My Cannabis & Motherhood certification was the first of its kind when it launch in August, 2018. We have doulas, doctors, nurses, moms, and budtenders taking the course. I've also recorded multiple courses for Green Flower Media as well as the Holistic Cannabis Academy on topics ranging from Cannabis and Mental Health, Cannabis and Women's Health to Cannabis as Preventative Medicine.

In 2013, I created a nonprofit called The Endocannabinoid Deficiency Foundation (THE ECDF) to drive clinical research, education, advocacy, and patient support on Cannabis for specific health conditions. In 2015, we changed the 501c3 nonprofit's name to IMPACT Network, and **IMPACT** Network's mission was **I**mproving **M**arijuana **P**olicy and **A**ccelerating **T**herapeutics for women worldwide. We were the first nonprofit to focus on Cannabis and women's health but closed in 2018 as the regulatory environment changed.

In 2017, I created Infused Health, which is an online platform that matches clients with clinicians using plant-assisted therapies (PAT) including Cannabis and mushrooms. Clients are paired with a vetted clinician that is experienced in using PAT for their health condition and is located in their city or state. This ensures that clients will get product and dosage recommendations that are safe, effective, affordable, and available in their location. We offer telehealth sessions, online courses, books, and products for every clients' budget.

I've been active in drug policy reform for Cannabis, kratom, and mushrooms including:

- Co-founder of Decriminalize Denver, the campaign that decriminalized "magic mushrooms" in Denver, the first city in the United States to do so (https://decriminalizedenver.org/).
- Research Director at Decriminalize California, the 2020 California state initiative (https://decrimca.org).
- Worked with the American Kratom Association to stop the DEA from placing kratom, a natural plant medicine with no overdose potential, as a Schedule 1 drug.
- Worked to add numerous qualifying conditions for medical marijuana cards in Colorado, Minnesota, Maine, and many other states.
- Worked to help legalize medical Cannabis in numerous states and countries and was a Drug Policy Alliance Partner.

I'm an advisor to several Cannabis companies, including:

- MyJane a subscription Cannabis for women (www.myjane.com),
- Mommy Complex (www.mommycomplex.com) which is a CBD line by moms for moms,
- Veda Warrior which is the first CBD line customized for your Ayurvedic dosha (www.vedawarrior.com),
- NanoSphere Health Sciences which produces Evolve Formulas Nanoserum which is a transdermal Cannabis gel pen (www.nanospherehealth.com)

I am also President of This is Jane Project, a nonprofit that supports women healing from trauma with Cannabis. I prefer to work with women-led companies in the Cannabis space or companies that give back to nonprofits or social justice initiatives in some way, although I also sit on all-male boards to ensure the female voice is represented.

118 · DR. MICHELLE ROSS

What are the misconceptions of Cannabis?

There are so many misconceptions about Cannabis. What's the most sad to me is I've met doctors, scientists, lawyers, and other highly educated professionals that have access to the same facts I do, but stigma or money causes them to ignore the medical benefits of Cannabis and, the devastation the war on drugs has done to communities of color.

For example, a large part of my work has been outreach to the medical and scientific community. In response, I've received detailed emails from Harvard doctors that my work advocating for mothers to use Cannabis is causing massive brain damage and birth defects and I should be thrown in jail. Needless to say, I haven't stopped educating mothers and I have an online certification on Cannabis and Motherhood for clinicians (www.Cannabisandmotherhood.com/course).

In multiple states, I've witnessed psychiatrists attend hearings for expanding qualifying conditions of medical marijuana cards to warn about the horrors of Cannabis. These psychiatrists are often paid by pharmaceutical companies that produce psychiatric medications that are threatened by the emerging Cannabis industry. Sadly, their testimony, no matter how outrageous or exaggerated, is viewed as credible by legislators and can block legislation including PTSD as a qualifying condition for medical marijuana for veterans. That's why it's so important for Cannabis doctors, scientists, and nurses to attend hearings and advocate for Cannabis patients.

When most people hear the term "Cannabis," they think of Marijuana and getting high when in fact Tetrahydrocannabinol (THC), the cannabinoid that gives user a euphoric feeling or "high," is just one of over 100 cannabinoids identified in the Cannabis sativa plant. As more and more research is conducted, scientists are finding tremendous therapeutic benefits using different combinations of cannabinoids.

What are the five questions you are most frequently asked?

1. Is CBD safe for pregnant or breastfeeding moms?

While more human research would be appreciated, both anecdotal evidence and preclinical research suggest minimal harm if any from using CBD while pregnant or breastfeeding. CBD does cross the placenta and is also excreted into breast milk, but little is actually passed from mother to child. CBD, because of its neurogenic and antioxidant properties is less likely to negatively impact a baby than THC.

CBD would be categorized as FDA Pregnancy Risk C, similar to THC, because it lacks clinical trials in pregnant women on its safety and efficacy and lacks clinical or rodent research suggesting it causes harm or birth defects. In fact, Epidiolex, a Schedule 5 CBD drug made by GW Pharma, asks pregnant women who use Epidiolex to register in order to track any adverse reactions in mother or baby. To give some context, there are drugs that are worse for pregnant women, Pregnancy Risk D, and Pregnancy Risk X (aka never, ever take).

2. Why doesn't my CBD oil work?

Patients often buy CBD online, at a gas station, or at a kiosk in the mall and don't know what to look for in a reputable brand, such as lab testing for heavy metals, pesticides, and solvents, or ingredients that are safe for human consumption. Some products have ZERO CBD or much less CBD than what is listed on the label. I make sure clients buy products that work, find their correct dosage, and if we still can't get there, then explore other pain relief options because for some patients, CBD alone is not enough.

3. Why do you charge for consultations?

Imagine going to your doctor, a specialist, who has spent years and hundreds of thousands of dollars on training, for a free appointment? For a consultation with a specialist, you usually pay twice as much as what you would with a primary care doctor.

A Cannabis coach, whether a doctor, nurse, certified health coach, or registered caregiver, is worth their weight in gold. Just because they are dispensing advice about Cannabis, and not a pharmaceutical drug, is not a reason to not pay them or to skip that process and seek out medical advice from a budtender. In some states, like Minnesota, Cannabis pharmacists determine which products and in what dosage you can buy, and you pick up your "prescription" at a dispensary and are not allowed to deviate. In Canada, Cannabis nurses provide these recommendations.

The Cannabis dispensary model in the United States is confusing to patients. Budtenders should be thought of as cashiers or pharmacists rather than medical professionals that can recommend products and dosages. In some states, such as Colorado, budtenders are banned from giving any medical recommendations and can only advise customers on smell, taste, and general effects.

You can consult Dr. Google for free, but of course, you get what you pay for. The internet is full of misinformation that could harm your health. You need to ensure Cannabis is right for you, won't interact with your current medications, and the product you are purchasing is safe to consume. When you pay for a Cannabis consultation, you are saving money in the long-term by avoiding purchasing the wrong products or products that could harm you. Finally, you are likely supporting a clinician that has spent years advocating for patients and lobbying for Cannabis legalization, unpaid.

4. How do you test for the endocannabinoid deficiency?

Endocannabinoid deficiency can feel a lot like burnout because the endocannabinoid system is often depleted when we are experiencing chronic stress. It would be great if there was a single biomarker we can test for, like there is with Vitamin D deficiency. Although my book is titled *Vitamin Weed: A 4-Step Plan to Prevent and Reverse Endocannabinoid Deficiency*, there is no "Vitamin Weed" to test for, as anandamide levels are just one piece of the picture.

The endocannabinoid system is complex (it is the largest neurotransmitter system in the body, after all). Endocannabinoid deficiency can be hard to test for because it can be local (for example, just in our brains or in our uteruses), or it can be throughout our body. A simple blood test can't get to the bottom of it, although in the future, we might be able to biopsy tissue or run an MRI to get the status of the cannabinoid receptor number or function.

Some DNA tests, like those offered by Endocanna Health (www.endocannahealth.com), are starting to look at mutations in our endocannabinoid system that could influence its function. For example, some people have a mutation in the FAAH, the enzyme that breaks down anandamide and makes it less functional. This results in an increase in anandamide (the same effect as if you were taking CBD). These patients are less likely to be endocannabinoid deficient and may even respond poorly to CBD or Cannabis treatment.

5. How can I find a doctor that is ok with my Cannabis use?

It is sometimes difficult to find a primary care doctor or specialist that supports Cannabis use. First, the doctors might not be educated about Cannabis and think it's harmful. Second, a doctor might think it's beneficial, but worry their employer or insurance provider will fire them for promoting Cannabis. Finally, the doctor might support Cannabis, but doesn't believe the products available in dispensaries are safe or effective.

Many patients believe they can go to any Cannabis doctor and get a treatment protocol that will help them with their medical condition. There's several problems with that assumption. Many Cannabis doctors just sign medical marijuana card paperwork, and you're in and out in five minutes. They legally can't, or just won't, tell you what products to take or what dosing is appropriate. Also, most Cannabis doctors were specialists before they became Cannabis doctors. So, a cardiologist that is now a Cannabis doctor isn't proficient on using Cannabis for every medical condition (and if they tell you they are, they are bluffing!).

What are the five questions people should be asking about Cannabis?

1. Is it safe to take CBD with my medication(s)?

If you're thinking about taking CBD while on other medications, take precautions. Unfortunately, CBD is a potent inhibitor of two types of p450 liver and gut enzymes (CYP3A4 and CYP2DC) that break down over one-third of prescription drugs. If you're using CBD with a drug that is metabolized by CYP3A4 or CYP2DC, the drug stays in your system longer. This can be dangerous because it could amplify the side effects of the drug like sleepiness, nausea, headache, blood thinning, or other serious issues. Many common drugs such as antidepressants, anti-seizure drugs, and blood thinners have reported interactions with CBD. Keep in mind that just because a drug has not had a published drug interaction, doesn't mean that is hasn't happened; it just means the research into it hasn't been funded.

I always recommend that patients on prescription medication talk with their doctor or other health professionals before using CBD, especially at doses higher than 10 milligrams of CBD per day. At Infused Health, we review a patient's medical history for potential drug interactions and then suggest that the dosage of medication be lowered (with their doctor's approval) or switch the patient to a different cannabinoid, such as THC, that doesn't have the same drug interaction.

2. **Is CBD or Cannabis right for me – or are there other plant-based medicines that might be better suited to treat my health issues?**

I think people need to look at all the tools in the toolbox. No treatment is right for everyone because we all have different genetics and levels of drug metabolism, and we experience different symptoms even with the same disease. CBD works differently than THC which works differently than kratom which works differently than medicinal and psilocybin mushrooms and so on. Each can target different neurotransmitter pathways.

For example, a patient with fibromyalgia might report CBD products don't help the pain and THC-containing Cannabis products increase the awareness of pain. That patient should be introduced to THCA which, unlike THC, doesn't cross the blood brain barrier but helps with inflammation and pain, kratom which activates the opioid system to relieve pain and fight fatigue, or mushrooms which can activate the serotonin system and help with pain and mood. Some patients align with one plant-based medicine while some use a combination on any given day.

I wish more clinicians were open to more than just Cannabis or pharma because there are more safe and effective options for patients. That's why I created the Institute of Plant-Assisted Therapy (IPAT) (www.ipatcertified.com) to train more clinicians in using Cannabis, mushrooms, kratom, and other plant-based medicines for healing emotional and physical pain.

3. How can I use Cannabis for my pain (and not just CBD isolate)?

Many people are scared of THC or smoking a CBD or Cannabis product. CBD oil or gummies sound innocent and safe, and don't come with that highly-stigmatized "high." But people don't realize that CBD is like Tylenol, whereas THC, or even THC + CBD is more like an oxycodone or stronger opioid. CBD doesn't work the same as THC. It merely increases levels of anandamide, our natural endocannabinoid, that bind to cannabinoid receptors much weaker than THC. THC binds strongly and decreases inflammation and pain and boosts mood much better than CBD alone. So, instead of constantly increasing the dose of your CBD-only product to no benefit, try adding some (or a lot) of THC to actually make a dent in severe pain.

4. How can I use Cannabis to heal rather than numb myself from emotional pain/trauma?

Cannabis, like any psychedelic is all about set and setting—where you are using it, who you are using it with, and why you are using it. What is your intention? To heal with Cannabis? To reprocess trauma and leave baggage behind? Or to numb yourself? To hide from a past that's too painful to deal with?

We tend to store pain in different parts of our body. You're likely going to store that trauma in your hip, neck, or back. If you don't deal with some of those emotional issues, you're never really going to get that pain out no matter how many opioids you use or how much Cannabis you smoke. It's mindset work. Cannabis, when used appropriately in a certain set and setting, can really help with trauma.

Cannabis stimulates your cannabinoid receptors which are found all over the body and brain. I did most of my research work on a region of the brain called the hippocampus that is important for learning and memory. When you stimulate your cannabinoid receptors, you're jumpstarting the circuitry that helps you forget – not helps you learn.

When thinking about trauma, think about what PTSD is. PTSD is characterized by people having nightmares, too many thoughts, and reliving their trauma. So, imagine if you could help somebody rewire their brain to forget or at least focus less on a horrible memory and let that go so they can move forward.

Healing happens if you can finally let go of that trauma and don't hurt so badly anymore. Your total stress levels would go down. Many of us are dealing with stress but we're not even conscious about it; it's in our subconscious. But we're constantly battling that stress and holding that in our body. When Cannabis is used with a proper mindset, and we connect with others instead of isolating ourselves, we can start to physiologically heal stress and trauma and physically heal pain.

I'm proud to be the President of the This is Jane Project (www.thisisjaneproject.com), a nonprofit dedicated to documenting and healing one million women with trauma through Cannabis and connection. Through sharing our stories with other women, we heal and break the stigma of using Cannabis instead of alcohol or antidepressants to cope. We have events around the country and are always looking for new hosts.

5. How do I find out what strain works for me, not what strain works for someone else?

Just like anti-depressants, there's no crystal ball to predict what product and what dosage will work for you. Cannabis is personalized medicine. I wish it was as simple as there's one strain for fibromyalgia, there's one for depression, and there's one for arthritis. The reality is, you could get 50 patients with fibromyalgia, give them 50 strains to test, and each person would prefer a different strain for their symptom management.

It's important for you to test as many products as possible. Keep a journal of what products you use, the symptom relief you get, and any side effects or notes (like you were 10x as active as you normally are, that day you thought the product didn't really work, etc.). This can be costly, so I suggest going to sample days at your local dispensary, trying and sharing products with friends, and ordering a subscription box like MyJane (www.myjane.com) that has smaller products to try out for each symptom (like sleep) saving you a lot of money.

What changes in the industry do you see coming in the future?

Federal legalization of Cannabis in some shape or form is coming within the next five years, with banking coming sooner than that. We'll see a flood of investment in the space as the risk and barriers to investing drop. Federal legalization may bring taxation and more regulation, and that means it will be more expensive to start or grow your Cannabis or CBD business.

Legalization also means brands could be sued for products that make consumers sick, or for bad information on Cannabis given by budtenders or Cannabis clinicians. A greater focus on risk management and compliance will be important.

I think that in five years, we're going to have a lot of the research published that people are working on now. Everything from Cannabis and pregnancy research to learning about what these minor cannabinoids like THCV do. I think that we're also going to be farther along with the science of how to produce these cannabinoids in yeast or bacteria and we're going to have a lot more rare cannabinoids at a lower point price.

After federal legalization, hospitals and universities will update their policies and adapt to this new legal system. Cannabis clinicians and even Cannabis might be covered by health insurance. I think our Cannabis industry will be thriving and coupled with the research, we'll be able to much more powerfully say, okay, Cannabis is very good for fibromyalgia. We know how to dose it, we know what products you need for it. Coupled with apps and artificial intelligence (AI), there will be a lot less guesswork and we might be able to say, "Here's your genetics. Here's what your medical history is. This is the exact cannabinoid products you need and the correct dose."

Give me an example for how Cannabis has been life changing for someone you know.

I've worked with thousands of Cannabis patients over the years so it's hard to just give one example. I met the most extraordinary young woman in my travels. Alexis Bortell was just nine years old when she was a speaker at the first Cannabis conference in Texas in 2015. She spoke about how she was having seizures all the time and missing school. Then her dad, who was a veteran, learned about Cannabis for PTSD as well as epilepsy. She began using Cannabis oil and hadn't had a single seizure in almost a year.

But the problem was she wasn't using CBD oil which was quasi-legal in Texas. She was using Cannabis oil that contained THC and CBD which was against the law in Texas. Alexis had to move to Colorado to be a legal medical marijuana patient, away from her friends and family, just so she could live seizure-free.

Alexis also spoke at my nonprofit's Cannabis & Brain Health Conference in 2016, and she blew everyone away. Little did I know this Cannabis advocate prodigy would go on to write a book and even sue Jeff Sessions and the United States government for keeping Cannabis a Schedule 1 drug despite its obvious medical value.

What do you wish people knew or understood about Cannabis?

I wish that people would stop demonizing THC-containing Cannabis products, especially for mental health. While THC at high doses on rare occasions can trigger psychosis in users that have mental health issues, it doesn't mean it's not safe or even beneficial when using the right product at the right dose. While I strongly suggest patients with schizophrenia or bipolar disorder first explore CBD under the care of an experienced Cannabis clinician (the potential for CBD to interact with medications for these disorders is high), the risk of exploring low-dose THC in other disorders is low.

Low-dose THC can be better at controlling anxiety or depression than CBD for some patients, as CBD may cause further depression of mood or irritability. THC brings mood up, whereas CBD can bring mood down. This makes sense when you think about someone with bipolar disorder. THC might trigger or worsen their mania, while CBD might help relax and level them out.

What are the most exciting cannabinoids?

There are over 111 cannabinoids, although only a few including CBD and THC are present in high enough amounts to have any clinical impact on our health. CBDA and THCA are the cannabinoids that are made in the hemp and Cannabis plants, and it take decarboxylating, or heating CBDA and THCA, to turn them into CBD and THC, respectively.

These "raw cannabinoids" act differently in the body and have different health benefits. CBDA, for example, is much better at lowering anxiety than CBD—at least in rodents. THCA doesn't cross the blood-brain barrier like THC, and only activates CB1 and CB2 receptors in the body, not the brain. THCA is a powerful anti-inflammatory (without the psychoactivity of THC) that is amazing for treating fibromyalgia, arthritis, lupus, and other conditions where inflammation is a primary driver of symptoms.

What is a Cannabis coach?

A Cannabis coach reviews your medical history, checks for potential drug interactions, discusses treatment goals, and identifies potential products and dosages to try. They help clients understand how to record their Cannabis experiences so they can identify what worked and what didn't work, how to navigate unwanted highs, and work with seriously ill patients on a regular basis.

Cannabis health coaches do not provide medical marijuana cards because they serve a transformational healthcare role, not a transactional role. In addition, not everyone needs a medical marijuana recommendation and a visit to a doctor or other qualifying practitioner. CBD products can be purchased online or in many stores without a card. Finally, many states and countries have legalized recreational marijuana and do not require customers to have a medical marijuana card to access Cannabis products containing THC.

You may have heard of Cannabis nurses. While some nurses (RNs) may have obtained additional Cannabis education, they are not the only qualified providers of Cannabis education and Cannabis health coaching. In fact, many qualified Cannabis health coaches in other fields do not have advanced degrees but have undergone rigorous training and are certified as health coaches through institutes like the Institute for Integrative Nutrition (INN) or the Holistic Cannabis Academy.

While some Cannabis coaches may have advanced degrees including MDs, DOs, NDs, PhDs, and RNs, they are not required to perform the role of Cannabis health coach. Advanced degrees are helpful for supervising other health coaches, consulting on medical conditions beyond wellness or pain management goals or being able to prescribe other prescriptions. I supervise the Cannabis health coaches at Infused Health. I have a PhD in Neuroscience and as a professor, I train Cannabis clinicians at several institutes including the Institute For Plant-Assisted Therapy (IPAT) and the Holistic Cannabis Academy.

Why is it important that someone talk to a Cannabis coach?

It's not as easy as smoke a joint and your pain will go away. Each patient has a unique medical history, genetics, liver, etc. that will require a different approach to Cannabis treatment. Invest in a Cannabis coach or Cannabis nurse to help you avoid wasting money on the wrong products, or worse, having to go to the ER because you experienced bad side effects, and get back to healthy faster.

Dr. Michelle Ross, PhD, MBA
Founder, Infused Health

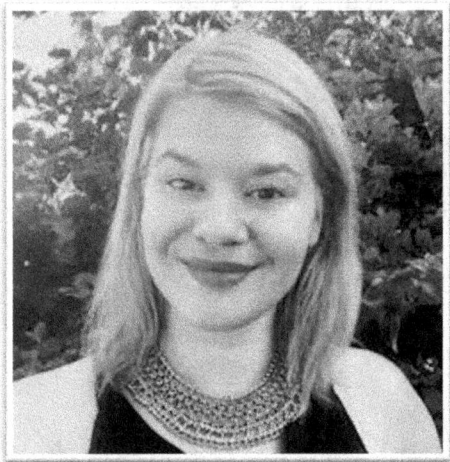

I'm a neuroscientist (aka brain scientist) who was diagnosed with fibromyalgia in early 2015 after battling blood clots in my lungs and legs, black mold poisoning, and lead poisoning. I went from wheelchair-bound and on tons of prescription drugs to traveling around the world living my best life all on plant medicine!

I help patients, healthcare professionals, and Cannabis industry professionals understand how to use Cannabis, CBD, kratom, and psilocybin mushrooms safely and effectively for themselves or their clients.

I'm an international speaker on Cannabis for women and have been helping patients with chronic illness thrive for the last seven years. I'm a scientist with a PhD in Neuroscience from the University of Texas Southwestern Medical Center at Dallas, where I studied in the department of Molecular Psychiatry.

I've written several best-selling books including *Vitamin Weed: A 4-Step Plan to Prevent and Reverse Endocannabinoid Deficiency* and *Train Your Brain to Get Thin: Prime Your Gray Cells For Weight*

Loss, Wellness, and Exercise. I'm also the CEO of Infused Health, a Cannabis health coaching platform.

I am a leader in the psilocybin mushroom decriminalization movement. I am currently the Research Director at Decriminalize California, the 2020 state initiative to decriminalize magic mushrooms, and was the co-founder of Decriminalize Denver, the successful May 2019 initiative, to decriminalize magic mushrooms in Denver, Colorado.

Fun fact: I was the first scientist to star on reality television 10 years ago on the hit CBS show *Big Brother*!

Rebekah Logie

When did your interest in Cannabis start and why?

One night in May 2014, I was asleep in my second story, one-bedroom apartment with my sweet chiweiner dog, Soco Baby. Soco began to growl and randomly bark, which he never does so I listened harder. I heard some commotion from my living room, so naturally, I got up to see what was going on.

When I walked into my living room, I saw my boyfriend whom I had broken up with four months prior. He had climbed onto my back screened-in balcony, slit the screen and entered my apartment through the sliding glass door. He immediately ran at me and grabbed me. He told me that if he couldn't have me, no one could. He threatened my life over and over saying, "You're going to die tonight!" and "No one will save you."

After three hours of fighting for my life and trying to escape my apartment, I finally was able to get him to leave. He took my laptop and phone so I wouldn't be able to call the police. Thank goodness I still had a phone and was able to call 911.

Fast forward six months later and after many trial dates, tears, confusion, and sleepless nights, I realized I was no longer mentally well. I began therapy and coping mechanisms, exercising more, and doing anything to help with my headspace. I had developed serious PTSD, anxiety, depression, and insomnia. Therapist after therapist wanted to prescribe every type of antidepressant (Xanax, Valium, etc.) I've never felt comfortable depending on a pharmaceutical, but I needed help.

The only natural thing that helped me sleep through the night terrors and helped motivate me to keep moving forward and not live life with a dark, depressed cloud over my head was Cannabis.

Thank goodness in 2016, Florida legalized medical Cannabis and I now had a new legal, holistic option available. This was life changing! I became a patient and learned so much more about Cannabis. I was obsessed with learning more about this miracle plant. I read any Cannabis book I could find from Jack Herer's *The Empower Wears No Clothes* to Lizzie Post's *Higher Etiquette*. (Two of my favorites — and if you haven't read them, please do!)

I learned about how CBD products could help with my anxiety and depression during the day without having to worry about the "euphoria" that comes with the higher THC products. I learned about the endocannabinoid system and the history of hemp and politics. I talked about Cannabis with anyone who would listen. I knew this was becoming a passion, and I wanted to help educate and inform people that this was an option that WORKED.

Cannabis works without killing your other organs and without risk of addiction. I began to seek employment opportunities in the Cannabis industry. I felt that would be the first step. I searched for weeks and applied to every position I saw available. One day, I saw a position in a dispensary nearby, and I knew I wanted this job. I emailed and called over, and over, and over, until someone finally returned my call.

I became a Wellness Coordinator (which is just a fancy name for their budtenders) for Surterra Wellness. I LOVED this job, LOVED! Being able to help patients find the perfect product for them was so exciting. I was able to teach them about how different terpenes, cannabinoids, and routes of administration can be beneficial to their ailments. Patients would come back after months of using Cannabis and would exclaim that they are completely off of their 20 different pills or that their condition had greatly improved or nearly disappeared. We had 2-year-old patients with epilepsy and 87-year-old grandmothers fighting cancer or extreme rheumatoid arthritis. Different ages, different conditions and each with their own medical Cannabis journey. It was an incredible experience and an opportunity I will never take for granted or forget.

I wanted to continue to do more and help more people learn that this was an option. So, I accepted a position as a Community Advocate. I was able to attend events and educate people about medical Cannabis and how to become a patient. I'm grateful for the opportunity to be able to help people learn and be a voice for this miracle plant. I will continue to break the stigma whenever and wherever I can.

What are the misconceptions of Cannabis?

- I often hear people say that Cannabis users are the typical lazy stoner, addicted to smoking weed while sitting on the couch and eating copious amounts of junk food. Cannabis makes people lazy or fat or unemployed. Wrong.
- Cannabis is addicting and is a gateway drug. Real Cannabis users will tell you that it is in fact the opposite of a gateway drug.
- Because it's a Schedule 1 drug, it must be as bad for you as meth. *eyeroll*
- Cannabis is for dirty hippies.
- Cannabis has no actual medicinal benefits.
- If Cannabis became legal, the crime rate would increase.
- CBD doesn't do anything for you; it's a placebo effect.

What questions are you most frequently asked?

- Will I become addicted to medical Cannabis?
- Will CBD make me high and unable to function?
- What are the medical benefits of Cannabis, both CBD and THC?
- Do I have to smoke it?

- Can I get fired from my job if I test positive for THC even though I am a patient?
- What questions should people be asking?
- Are my products good quality, full spectrum and do the manufacturers provide third-party testing results?
- Are higher CBD or higher THC products more beneficial for what I'm trying to treat?
- Which route of administration is the most effective for my ailment?
- Is there a particular terpene that can assist with my ailment?
- What is the onset period and duration of the product? Should I double up on routes of administration?

Give me a few examples of a positive experience, benefits, or success stories.

My favorite success story comes from a patient that I helped on her very first visit to the dispensary. She had recently received her approval email and was ready to try medical Cannabis. A friend had dropped her off, and when she walked in, I could tell she was heavily medicated.

I signed her in and then sat down to do a consultation with her. I asked a few questions and could tell she wasn't really following what I was trying to explain. Her eyes were barely open, and her head seemed heavy. We settled on a higher THC product because she was able to explain that she had chronic pain for which she had been taking high doses of morphine.

I finished going over instructions on how and when to use her product and her friend arrived to take her home.

One month later, the same women drove up on her motorcycle. She was completely cognizant and bright eyed and excited! She gave me the most sincere embrace and with tears in her eyes, she went on to tell me that she had been struggling with morphine and meth addiction and that she had planned to kill herself as an escape if she couldn't take control of her situation.

Using the products that she took home the previous month, she was able to completely quit abusing the drugs and detox herself back into a functioning human again. She explained that her husband had supported her and pushed her to try medical Cannabis as a last-ditch effort and she was so grateful that she tried it. She thanked me for being patient with her and helping her the best I could. Cannabis literally saved her life.

Most of my patients are, surprisingly, older females. Many of them are seeking relief from menopause, arthritis, cancer, or even depression. I've had some patients come in that are terrified to try Cannabis and are only trying because their child/spouse encouraged them to do so. They always ask the most questions and are very hesitant to believe in the products.

These patients are my favorite because 9 times out of 10, they return and are so excited to tell me how they've improved. I also love the patients that have doubting spouses. They will bring in their spouse to ask questions or to learn more about Cannabis that often they don't really care to learn. Weeks later, they return with praise about how their partner has improved that they've told everyone they know that Cannabis really works!

What is the recommended starting doses for clients? Can you overdose? What are the side effects?

I always explain the "start low and go slow" rule, especially for patients with no Cannabis experience. Wait 1.5-2 hours if ingesting and be very cautious when consuming Cannabis orally for the first few times. Since it's being broken down by the liver, it general takes much longer to activate, but can feel more intense.

You cannot overdose, but it is possible to consume an amount that makes you feel uncomfortable or too much of that euphoria.

When this happens, I recommend you have a CBD vape nearby to help counteract the high. If you don't have a CBD vape, chewing peppercorns can have the same reaction. (Gross, but it works!)

Worst case scenario, you can try to sleep it off and use a lesser amount next time. When you find your right dosing, your body will know. It can be a bit of trial and error in the beginning, so try to remain patient.

How was Cannabis life changing for someone you know?

Other than my personal experience, I've seen many patients have success and their Cannabis use has been life changing. One in particular that stands out is a patient that was suffering with severe Parkinson's. His condition became increasingly worse as he aged, and he could barely function due to extreme tremors. We tried a vape pen and within less than a minute, his tremors ceased. It was like watching a miracle happen. His hands became steady and he was able to calm down and relax. After about five minutes of him just sitting still, he reached over and was able to hold his wife's hand again *queue the tears*. He figured out a regimen that worked best for him and began to use the tincture for lasting relief and the vape for the mornings or if he had any breakthrough pain/tremors. He was able to hold his wife again; he was able to brush his teeth easily again. Cannabis gave him his independence back.

How has Cannabis helped you, your clients, or others where other products were unsuccessful?

Cannabis helps me relax when I start to feel overwhelmed or anxious. I prefer to use a high CBD vape during the day, and especially in those moments of anxiety. I suffer greatly from social anxiety, depression, and anxiety as a whole. Using that higher CBD helps me combat my mental fight and relax.

I can socialize and not stay in my own mind, worrying all the time. I enjoy using sativa strains for those mornings when getting up is difficult or when I just need an extra burst of creativity, but I have to be extremely careful not to consume too much because it can trigger anxiety sometimes more than it can help.

At night, I like to use higher THC, indica leaning products to assist with my sleeping and just to relax after a long day. Consuming high THC Cannabis at night helps me deal with my PTSD and insomnia. In the past, when I would finally fall asleep after tossing and turning for many hours, I would wake up with night terrors or terrible episodes of sleep paralysis. Using Cannabis before I go to sleep helps me fall asleep faster and stay asleep without the terrors/paralysis. I can actually get eight uninterrupted hours of sleep.

Before I became a patient, I had read about CBD chews that were supposed to help with anxiety and depression. After spending (too much) money on these chews, I was so excited to give them a try. They. Did. Nothing. I was so disappointed and didn't want to invest any more money in Cannabis products. After researching more and learning the differences between hemp and CBD, I learned that the particular chews I had purchased were just hemp chews with very little health benefits for what I was battling. I also try to explain to my patients the difference between hemp, full spectrum CBD, and broad-spectrum CBD.

What changes in the industry do you foresee coming in the future?

I believe that as more research occurs and as we are able to conduct more studies, we will learn even more about the benefits of this plant. I'd love to see the discovery of new cannabinoids and terpenes or how different combinations can help exact conditions. I see the industry moving quickly once it becomes federally legal with possible new routes of administration that could be even more health conscious. I foresee Cannabis becoming the norm and a first option, and not as a last resort. I imagine that dispensaries will be as popular as your well-known drugstores and convenience stores. I hope that Cannabis can be spoken about open and freely.

What do you wish people knew or understood about Cannabis?

That this is a plant. This is a medicine. This isn't some addicting, scary drug. I wish people knew how people benefit from it and that it saves lives. I would love to invite any person who is skeptical to spend one day in a dispensary and listen to stories of our patients that come in. We need to fight the stigma that was created to line politician's pockets. Cannabis is the future of natural healing and we need to embrace that now.

What is important to look for when selecting a Cannabis product?

Things to consider when selecting a Cannabis product:

- Route of Administration – vaping, oral ingesting, smoking, topical, suppository, or edibles. Which method works best for your goals?
- CBD Content – Are you fighting inflammation, anxiety, depression? Do you need higher CBD products? Do you need a specific ratio of CBD:THC?
- THC Content – Are you in chronic pain or do you need assistance with sleep or appetite? Do you need just THC with little to no CBD?
- Third-Party Testing – Are the results of each product available and acceptable?
- Price – Does it fit your budget long term? Can you find a more affordable product?

- Quantity – Depending on your consumption, should you make one large purchase or multiple smaller purchase?
- Availability – Will this product continue to be available?

You have had such a powerful and resilient life, what message would you like to give cancer patients about the usage of Cannabis?

Stay strong. You have a community behind you that is supporting you whether you're aware of it or not. Don't get discouraged if someone judges or doesn't understand your healing process. Read more Cannabis books, do a lot of research for yourself. Surround yourself with people who do care and encourage your Cannabis journey through recovery. You've got this.

I honor your knowledge and advocacy regarding Cannabis. What changes in public education of Cannabis can we start with today?

Providing more free, educational programs are a great and easy start. I've attended many of these events and they've always had a great turn out. Most people just want the opportunity to learn without any obligations to make purchases or requirements to see a doctor. Virtual and anonymous consultations should be made available for people that may still feel uncomfortable about discussing Cannabis.

Also, normalizing Cannabis and openly speaking about the benefits of Cannabis or the latest news about Cannabis. Let's make Cannabis a widely spoken topic of conversation. Discuss with your children and explain to the younger generation the positives and benefits of Cannabis.

Your passion about Cannabis is so contagious. How can we provide the public a guideline for buying the best products and avoiding the bad stuff out there?

Third-party testing! Be sure you know what's in your products. Spend some extra time researching and ensuring the company and its products are legitimate. Ask for recommendations from credible sources. Don't just purchase the cheapest option from a gas station. Sometimes, you get what you pay for, and when it's something you're putting in your body – you don't want cheap.

CBD for Wellness:

Did you know that your body produces natural cannabinoids? These endocannabinoids interact with your endocannabinoid System (ECS). This newly-discovered system works to keep all of your other systems balanced. The ECS is made up of a series of cannabinoid receptors throughout your entire body, including your brain, organs, connective tissues, and more.

While your body produces endocannabinoids, sometimes you can experience endocannabinoid deficiency. This can even be in the form of a migraine, fibromyalgia, and other symptoms. Using CBD and Cannabis can help by adding phyto-cannabinoids that your body receives just like endocannabinoids! Consider cannabinoids like any other nutrient your body needs. When your body is lacking iron, you can take iron supplements. When your body is lacking cannabinoids, you can consume Cannabis. I am a strong believer in using CBD daily, like a multivitamin.

Approaching an older family member about CBD:

Approaching a family member about using CBD can be a tricky topic depending on their background and their beliefs of Cannabis. Some of our older relatives were raised during the "Reefer Madness" and "Just Say No" era, so they may be hesitant or just not interested at all. This can provide a challenging predicament when trying to help, if that's the case. Be respectful and understanding when you're explaining why CBD could be beneficial for them. Breaking the stigma requires education and compassion.

I feel that since it's recently become a hot topic and it's more openly discussed, people are becoming more accepting and even curious about CBD. Hopefully, this will continue in the future and no one will need to have that uncomfortable talk.

Regardless of their mentality towards Cannabis, if you think they could benefit from CBD, definitely bring it up. I like to explain how CBD and THC differ and in what ways each cannabinoid can be beneficial. I always make sure to really explain how CBD can benefit their specific condition and I try to find other examples/testimonials about the same condition and their improvements once using CBD.

Another important thing to explain is the different routes of administration. Users don't need to know how to roll a joint and smoke it; they can simply drop some tincture in their tea. Nice and easy. I recommend smaller doses in an easy-to-measure form (tinctures or capsules) for a beginner, and as always, go low and slow. If they try it for two weeks and don't feel a change, increase the dosage. I also recommend keeping a wellness journal, especially in the beginning. This can be a helpful tool to track the dose taken, onset time and the benefits or side effects felt.

Be especially patient with their questions and spend as much time as needed to ensure they fully understand how to dose and administer their CBD. If used incorrectly, they could become easily discouraged and quit before they find their "sweet spot" (my version of the point when a patient has found the perfect dosage to reach the maximum potential of the CBD in their system). Remember, every person is different, each experience will differ, and not everyone will react the same.

About Rebekah Logie

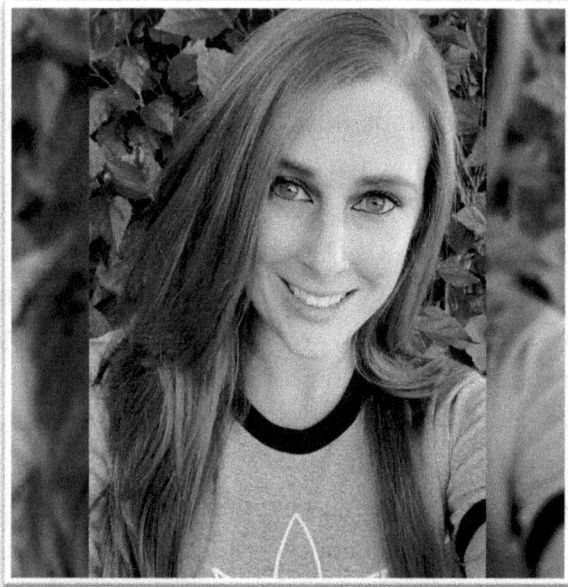

Rebekah Logie was born in Tampa, FL and raised in North Carolina. After a few adult years in NC, she decided that the Sunshine State was calling her name again. Chasing her dream of working with marine animals at Seaworld, she found herself in Orlando. Little did she know that Cannabis would soon become her passion.

When she isn't advocating for Cannabis within the community, she loves spending time with her family and three fur babies. They often frequent the nearby theme parks and enjoy being in the sunshine. Her favorite hobbies include reading books about Cannabis, going to the beach or hiking Florida nature trails.

Stephanie Johnson

Tell me about your journey with Cannabis. What is your area of expertise?

I'm a Cannabis late bloomer compared to so many others deep in the industry. I was a "Gen X, DARE Generation" kid who always complied with Nancy's directive to "Just Say No." It wasn't until I was 38 years old and diagnosed with an aggressive breast cancer known as Triple Negative Invasive Ductal Carcinoma that I had seriously entertained Cannabis. I was found to be in Stage 3, Grade 3, and BRCA1 positive; which meant that I had the gene abnormality - the only thing I'll ever have in common with Angelina Jolie (except, maybe, the tattoos). That would affect my treatment plan, the number of surgeries needed, and my survival rate. At the time, it was looking like I had less than a 25% chance to see five years. My children were still in high school. I wanted to hedge my bets and Cannabis had a lot of great points in its favor.

I had always been a researcher with over a decade in the world of media and communications. I was not afraid to hunt for truths, and this subject was no exception. I read citable study after study; Cannabis as a whole, Cannabis and cancer, Cannabis and triple negative breast cancer. It was researched, read and questioned.

On the day of my first visit to my oncologist – a heavily experienced breast oncologist – I was sure to ask his opinion. I do remember how it had made me a bit sad that he had to restrict how he could speak on the subject due to existing laws. He did say that if I chose to consume, then I was to keep him informed as we were on the same team – to which I agreed. He assured me no one would tell me I couldn't.

I coupled that with my pile of information and I was as ready as I could ever be. It helped me navigate, in great ways, through the toughest year of my life.

Since then, Cannabis-based products have been a part of my daily life. Personally – for residuals from that year of fighting cancer (neuropathy, etc.) but also because I truly believe in the plant's capacity against many forms of breast cancer – or what many studies have shown.

While there are still days in which I find myself marveling at the ability to speak so candidly on it – and in so many ways – I am also excited to be a part of it. I am especially grateful because my experience brought me here in a truly experiential way – and a way that many could attest to. It is exciting to be a part of Cannabis right now.

In addition to this personal experience, I am able to work within the space, daily, at an advertising, marketing and branding firm in Dallas, Texas. My experience in journalism, research, and copywriting is utilized in multiple ways. I am part of a creative and communications team – a group of us who work together from research to content. I am the Senior Communications Strategist, essentially meaning if there are words required, I'm probably nearby. I'm also a licensed and trained cosmetologist and cosmetology educator. I'm very passionate about the merge of CBD into the world of lifestyle and beauty – especially skin and hair.

Many of our clients are either CBD, hemp, Cannabis, fitness, or food & beverage brands. This gives me a great scope of opportunities in the industry. It fits well with my experience and my natural inclination to mine for information. We're given a lot of opportunities to blend the need for well-researched content and creativity, together, and it's a lot of fun for me. We have multiple offices and have growth into places like Latin America – it's exciting to be a part of it. I'm glad to get to do it.

When did your interest in Cannabis start and why? Why did you start your business?

My main interest developed when I got sick with cancer. I think that's a more common tale than not.

I wouldn't say I'm a completely independent business since I work at The Skyline Agency. I still do some freelance work and write some journalistic copy for places like Benzinga. I think that it is important that we have the conversation and that we're not scared of it. We must ensure we're putting out good information, being mindful of those who aren't yet in the know, and always desirous of doing our best work that moves the industry forward.

What are the misconceptions of Cannabis?

Common misconceptions include:

- Cannabis is "marijuana."
- That it is dangerous.
- That it is lethal.
- That it makes you crazy or unmotivated or misanthropic.

This plant is straight from the ground and has myriad uses. It's mind-boggling to me that it is classified, federally, as it is. We need to federally legalize it so we can accurately and comprehensively have open studies and conversations about it.

Misconceptions about hemp, the federally legal cousin of marijuana that the bulk of CBD products are coming from, these days:

- It is the same thing as marijuana (it is not)
- That it can get you "high"

Hemp is, in my opinion, highly underrated. It has thousands – THOUSANDS – of uses. It is so much more than CBD – fuels, textiles, papers, hempcrete… nearly endless. I'm a big fan of hemp.

I truly believe that hemp is a plant that should be utilized more and not just within the CBD space. I think that it's a plant that is good for many uses but also good for American farmers. I would like to see more Whole Hemp discussions – talking on creating partnerships between spaces in the hemp industry – and growing it all for the betterment of everyone involved.

What questions are you most frequently asked?

"Is hemp the same as marijuana?" – This may seem like a basic question to a lot of us who do read and write about the subject every day, but I believe many still don't know. It's a phrase that is commonly trending. There's a reason it keeps coming up. Other very common plant and compound-related questions are: "Does CBD get you high?", "Is CBD weed?"

"Do you get weed at work?" – There are those questions that have the assumption behind them that those who work in the industry are all just sitting around in a smoke-filled conference room and watching Netflix. It's the same vein as those who think Cannabis makes people lazy. I know we're very committed and professional, just as many who are in the industry.

"Is it hard to get into the industry?" – I think that it may require a bit more networking in some areas, but, like any industry, bring good work. Naturally, it's easier to find jobs in the industry when in a legal state – as there are more employment opportunities as a whole – but there are jobs out there. I find that this is a great market for creatives, developers, and other professionals like ours because of the rapid growth of the industry. The longevity of any company in this industry is going to be dependent on having great talent, great resources, authenticity and an ability to ride out a wave of activity for a while.

"Do you have to participate to work in it?" – I don't think so. There are plenty of people that work in the space who are not consumers, and that's okay. You don't have to consume products to be good at writing code or editing high quality video.

"Is it difficult being a woman in Cannabis?" – I have not had a negative experience to speak of. I have heard of some who have, but I've been fortunate to not have to experience that. I think, too, because I'm on a more creative, research and content side, we are keyboard bound for most of our time.

What questions should people be asking?

People need to really be asking their representatives why this isn't completely legal yet because we're hindering ourselves by being this way. We're beyond the old stories. We can just be open and candid about it.

I would like to see more people talking about the business of hemp and Cannabis and how it can be great for farming and agricultural communities. I grew up in the central states so my heart is always in Nebraska. I think this plant can be great for them. There should be more queries about the possibilities and uses, too, so that these farmers are shown the hope that comes with the crop. Yes, of course in CBD and the cannabinoids that can be extracted, but also the husks and seeds. Every part of the plant has potential, and that is a story worth telling.

Let's talk about the ancillary services and the jobs that the industry creates. Let's talk about the good environmental impacts of hemp.

Give me a few examples of a positive experience, benefits, or success stories.

Personally – for me – it got me through cancer, first, and life, since. I currently enjoy utilizing topicals for my continued neuropathic – cancer related – issues in my feet and hands. Ingested, Cannabis-related products help me with my appetite, digestion, and feeling of regularity and balance in my system. It helps me rest and sleep. I'm not a physician, but this is my personal experience. I also have a dog who's a rescue and has moments when he cannot "deal" (thunderstorms, etc.) – where a little doggie CBD treat helps him to cope. He's 12 now so I think he's earned his right to relax.

My sister had also changed her opinions of Cannabis over the years. Her own daughter – my niece – works in the industry in Colorado Springs. She's worked at the dispensary level and has recently worked creating graphics and is looking into growing into the content space herself.

I love being able to change perceptions on an individual level – conversation by conversation. Not all are winners, mind you, but it's always refreshing to hear other's similar tales.

I write a lot about my own experiences and contribute to stories about breast cancer survivorship so, over the years, some readers have found me on Twitter and have directed questions at me because someone in their life has been diagnosed with breast cancer. I try to be candid and keep sharing what I know and hope that they all have successful outcomes.

Recommended starting doses for clients? Can you overdose and what are the side effects?

From what I understand, it is physically impossible to overdose from Cannabis. I've read that even if you – somehow – could consume hundreds of pounds at once (not likely) that it still wouldn't be enough. Surely, hemp won't do it, but even though many have told tales of edibles "sneaking up on them," I've only known of a long nap and a desire for snacks as being the main downfall.

When people ask me about serving sizes of CBD, or adding CBD to their lifestyle or wellness routine, I recommend everyone start small and work their way up in dosage until they feel it is effective. Most will say to begin at 20 mg per day and increase in increments of 5 mg until that desired result is achieved. It is good to research your manufacturer's instructions and literature, too.

If you're unsure or just want to try it on that "achy shoulder," starting with a topical product is a great way to be introduced.

How was CBD life changing for someone you know?

I have a pal who is a very hard working performer and beauty professional, and the addition of CBD to her life has been beneficial. She had recently stated that she's felt it has made great contributions in body aches and general stress and anxiety.

There are some great blogs out there like "The Lady Jane Project" that catalog these real-life stories for people to be able to research and read. More women like myself are sharing more, too.

How has CBD helped you/clients/others where other products were unsuccessful?

For me, it was about what I wanted to be working with for many years of my life. Did I want to take several anti-inflammatory pills – every day for years – and take on those tested risks with my body having had enough chemistry for one lifetime or, have a solution with much smaller – minimal – risk with the desired benefits? It's also about "hedging my bets." I don't believe it's a cure-all. I think it's scientifically inappropriate to say that about anything in the world, but I do believe that it has many more benefits than downfalls. It just so happens that it's many benefits align with my needs.

What changes in the industry do you foresee coming in the future? For legal issues as well as a consumer viewpoint.

I think that more states will come on board. It's bound to happen – no one wants to be the odd man out. I hope to see a true federal legalization in my lifetime, but we'll see.

Right now, it depends on the FDA rulings and how CBD will potentially be classified.

I think many minds are learning and changing, though. I see more people being okay with talking about Cannabis or aligning with it. The company, Edible Arrangements, has an edible CBD line now. There's still some evolution as a whole but I think that more products are to come.

I also think that the beauty space has just hit the tip of the iceberg on what CBD will be in and can potentially do. The studies regarding how CBD helps skin – especially with those who have issues like eczema and psoriasis – are inspiring.

What do you wish people knew or understood about CBD?

That it is just one little part of a big plant of beneficial compounds, and this is not just a fad that's going away any time soon. Will the industry evolve more? Surely, and in exciting ways, so get to know it more. You might be pleasantly surprised.

What is important to look for when selecting a CBD product ?

Research the company that is manufacturing your product. Their website should contain information from their hemp farm to their extraction process. They should absolutely have their

Certificates of Authenticity available for review. Some companies will have QR codes on their packaging that will link to their certificates while others have them on their website exclusively.

Be sure to read the label on the front and back – especially ingredients. For example, hempseed oil is not CBD. Don't buy something that isn't correct. If you're looking for CBD, it will say CBD or cannabidiol in the ingredients. A little due diligence goes a long way.

I also think it's good to be sure to chat with your doctor before you begin enjoying CBD products – especially if you're currently taking any medications. Just as you wouldn't want to have wine or beer with some medications, I believe in being candid and forthcoming with our medical professionals for our own safety.

Are there any questions that you feel you would like to address that were not asked?

I think it is important for people to talk about how this is not a typical industry or business or start up. Anyone wanting to get into and survive this space will need more than just a lot of money; they'll need experienced partners and professionals. Without people who understand FDA regulations and terminology, what the FTC expects all while navigating how to be seen among the masses, it's going to be really tough to survive. People with industry know-how and proven results are needed more than ever.

I honor your knowledge and advocacy regarding Cannabis. What change in the education of the public in terms of Cannabis can we start with today?

This book is a great way – gathering insight and hosting conversations is always a good idea. Knowledge is power, no matter the subject. I think we need to agree on our terminology as much of the public is confused about the differences between marijuana and hemp.

We have to agree that we can't expect people to research and come to us, so we need quality advocacy throughout the media landscape and in multiple forms.

In the beauty industry, product lines have educators and product/brand specialists that purely share information. They teach the practitioners and the publics. I would like to see more of this. I would like to see more of a push toward that experiential educational marketing.

Your passion about Cannabis is so contagious. How can we make sure we provide the public a guideline on buying the best products and avoiding the bad stuff out there?

Research – Research – Research! Reputable companies are transparent about their practices and their product. Look for true seed-to-sale providers who operate under regulatory bodies. Those who are compliant aren't afraid to tell you about it. Cheaper is not always going to be better. Quality product and quality extraction can be expensive. Read your labels.

How does CBD fit into the beauty industry?

It's the next big beauty gamechanger. It's going to be everywhere and in so many items - especially skin care. The studies I've been reading regarding what CBD does in the skin, for the homeostasis and redox balance, is really exciting. I'd say to keep an eye out because we've only just begun in beauty.

How is CBD different from other products? What are the benefits?

The studies on CBD and the skin – as I had stated above – are really exciting. There have been numerous reports executed that have shown the anti-inflammatory properties of CBD in the skin and how it has positive benefits for those who are dealing with things like eczema, psoriasis, and inflammatory acne. It also has incredible antioxidant power and there's been many positive results in how it fights UV damage and photoaging.

There are going to be a lot of people who will be very excited, I believe, to see this segment grow. I know I'm one of them.

Do you recommend any specific products?

Currently, the beauty market is still growing, but I've enjoyed the Cannuka body butter – it's great for the severely dry, cracked skin. It's very dense so you'll want to warm it in your palm to emulsify it. A little goes a long way.

In standard topicals, Medterra Rapid Cooling Cream 750 mg is a great choice for my neuropathy. I also like We Heart CBD body oil with patchouli – great for at night and for sore legs.

How do you use these products with your clients?

I don't service clients directly; my beauty knowledge is for the research and development of beauty products that I do with my work at the agency. I have practical experience in the field but dedicate all of my expertise to the development and accurate branding of CBD-based beauty that we work with.

Are some types of beauty products and CBD better than others?

There aren't enough product types out there to make an accurate comparison, but I think skin care is going to be the biggest segment to enjoy the benefits of adding CBD to their products – or creating new SKUS with it. I envision foundation will soon follow.

Lotions and body oils are also great because of the hydrating nature of the compound and the ease in which it works with similar foundations.

About Stephanie Johnson

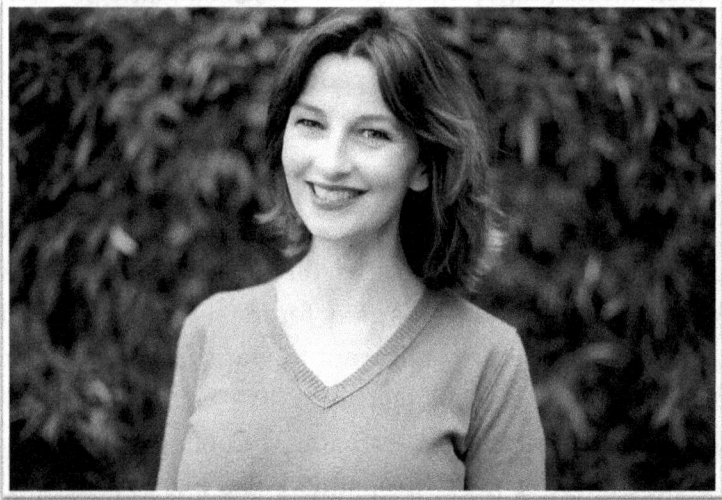

Stephanie Johnson is a research and communications professional for The Skyline Agency in Dallas, Texas where she utilizes her skill set to further conversations in areas of beauty, lifestyle, Cannabis, and wellness.

She has nearly two decades of experience in writing, journalism, broadcasting, and media management. An advocate, she regularly speaks on breast cancer survivorship and is not afraid to be candid for initiatives that are close to her heart.

Veronica Mitchell

What is your experience with Cannabis and your area of expertise?

I'm a writer and consultant working with seniors, Cannabis companies, and caregivers. I was the founder of two corporations, one of them being a senior's services and transportation business in San Diego. I have worked with the aging population in San Diego for more than 15 years. I continue to serve on various committees and volunteer with organizations serving seniors and caregivers throughout San Diego, CA. Speaking engagements fill my calendar throughout the year, which allows me to see the Cannabis industry and seniors in other cities.

I knew my next venture would have to find an avenue to combine my love of tech, business, Cannabis, and wellness. With Cannabis becoming a legal, history-making industry, and science starting to support many of the medicinal aspects of this plant, I decided to come out of the "Cannabis closet" on LinkedIn and started making connections in the industry.

I found a way to combine several passions of mine: advocating for seniors and women, writing and public speaking, business, and Cannabis medicine. I have 30 years of experience regularly consuming Cannabis as a patient. For the last five years, I have been researching Cannabis and writing about many areas of the Cannabis industry from medical technology and science research to products and brands. My ongoing education and research added to my real-life experience and ability to work with the medical community have positioned me to provide trusted, valuable information to the public.

Helping caregivers, seniors, their families, and medical teams navigate this new legal Cannabis industry is challenging and rewarding. All of what I do is my small part in normalizing Cannabis medicine and wellness for mainstream America so they will just consider Cannabis as an option for their aging care plans.

"It's always a process with all new Cannabis users and especially so with boomers, seniors, and caregivers because you have to hurdle the "drug stigma" until you reach the other side to acceptance of plant medicine." – Veronica Mitchell

For years, I have been a member of committees and have volunteered with organizations that have a mission to improve the lives of seniors and caregivers. I am passionate about bringing my Cannabis work into these committees that include business owners, government agencies, non-profits, and corporations, because it brings awareness to the importance of a legal Cannabis industry. For me, it's crucial to be of service to these communities. Whether I'm making introductions or speaking at events, together it bridges the gap and creates dialogue demonstrating that the Cannabis industry is professional and has a place in our community development and outreach.

Cannabis education is important for this writer and consultant because there is real research being conducted and, with federal legalization on the horizon, there will be much more scientific and medical research. Scientists are doing more and more studies on the plant as legal Cannabis keeps growing. Learning about the plant is crucial for me because I want to revise my aging plan and adjust it as I discover better options for my healthcare.

I've been educating and assisting my 85-year-old parents with Cannabis medicine for the first time in their lives. Both my parents have serious medical conditions, so navigating their proper dosages, delivery systems, brands, and products that work for individual biochemistry is critical for their overall health. I revisit and adjust their Cannabis plans as needed.

All older adults should be cautious when beginning their Cannabis consumption because it's not just for laughs as some advertisements might suggest. There are serious health risks for some seniors because of potentially critical health complications. All this needs to be considered and addressed with family, care teams, and medical professionals before the senior purchases Cannabis and CBD. The elderly typically have compromised immune systems, balance issues, bowel and gut challenges to mention but a few. There are also risks for drug interactions and allergies. It's just not as simple as let's go get Cannabis for grandma and grandpa. Cannabis is a very seemingly safe option for seniors but always use with care and caution.

I'm grateful to be a pioneer assisting the industry, my parents and their friends, and so many others understand that Cannabis can be a very safe option for seniors and caregivers. The last five years of my Cannabis research and work with my parents have been invaluable and instrumental in moving my career into being a leader in the Cannabis industry for trauma recovery, seniors and caregivers. We now have science, facts, research, and an actual legitimate industry.

I consult with families and seniors to help them discover the facts and science of Cannabis along with all the new technology being developed in this fascinating industry. Senior living communities consult with me for Cannabis educational events, awareness, and vetting organizations. Cannabis brands and companies consult with me to learn how to reach senior consumers and their loved ones. As a writer, I'm a columnist ("Ask Veronica") for the San Diego Union-Tribune, I write for various media outlets on a wide range of Cannabis topics, as well as writing guest blogs, advertorials, content, and white papers for various Cannabis companies.

When did your interest in Cannabis start and why?

I've been using Cannabis since my late teens. After I tried it with friends, I realized almost immediately that it was helping me. I didn't know anything about the plant because it was not presented as a medicinal experience – it was about experimenting and having fun with friends.

At that time, I had no education in Cannabis and there was little discussion about Cannabis other than it was a bad drug like heroin or cocaine. Yet, intuitively, I knew it was working medicinally in my body and wanted to keep using it. I needed to explore and research for myself if this new "drug," Cannabis, was benefitting me. Let me explain. I was a victim of childhood sexual abuse, and in my late teens, I had lots of trauma to heal. I discovered that when I smoked Cannabis it relaxed me, my mind, and my body which I desperately needed. I lived in fear and was never able to get good sleep, so Cannabis provided relief and that helped me heal and move forward in life. In those days, there wasn't much discussion about healing from childhood sexual abuse, and I found that a little bit of Cannabis provided hours of relief and relaxation which gave me the ability to function with less fear and anxiety. I had to figure it out and find a way to continue using it.

For my friends it was more of, "we'll try it again, no big deal." For me, I remember feeling calmer and not obsessing on the abuse and trauma which was a game-changer for me. My childhood sexual assault had ended and this was years after it happened, so being able to get a moment to rest in thoughts or relax enough to have fun "in the moment" or enjoy a run without all the fearful thoughts was incredible to me. I instinctively knew that I had to use this type of "medicine" or alternative/natural help. By 20, I was seeing a Chinese Medicine Doctor and Naturopath doctor in addition to my "regular" medical team, so experimenting with natural health and plant-based medicine was part of my progression of using Cannabis and other alternative measures for good mind-body healthcare.

How did you start working in the Cannabis industry?

My passion for business and watching the Cannabis industry start sprouting up in states where it's legal got me thinking that I wanted to be involved in the fastest-growing, history-making industry. So, I started connecting with Cannabis companies on LinkedIn and other social media platforms. There I could make comments and start growing my knowledge base. I used social media and networking to increase my education and visibility in the industry. I started attending events and networking to find sources and companies that I could profile or guest blog. These were all efforts to leverage my education, network, and experience to find a career path in the industry.

It turns out, I had the best entry for myself and where I want to take my career. I stayed in my lane of seniors and caregivers and added my passion and knowledge of Cannabis into the mix. I started attending science and medical Cannabis conferences and working with my parents' healthcare professionals. All the while, continuing my same work with all the committees and organizations that I had been working with in San Diego for 15 years. Now, I just include my Cannabis consulting and speaking career. My hesitation quickly washed away because there were so many colleagues and associates that were curious or had a client or loved-one that was seeking Cannabis information so it was an easier transition than I had anticipated.

I work with seniors and caregivers because I know Cannabis can improve or alleviate some health conditions in both demographics. For seniors, it can help them with so many age-related conditions from arthritis to anxiety to better sleep and gut issues, so it makes sense if it's done safely and in conjunction with existing medical professionals. For caregivers that can legally consume Cannabis without jeopardizing their employment, it can offer better sleep, reduced stress and anxiety, and relieve muscle aches and pains. For both seniors and caregivers, these groups suffer higher rates of stress, depression, and isolation. Many turn to alcohol to ease their frustrations and loneliness. Using alcohol to ease stress is not healthy and increases other health ailments for many older adults and caregivers. For these same groups, Cannabis often proves to be a safer and healthier option for not only stress management but also when celebrating, without the hangover from alcohol.

Many medical professionals are starting to accept and acknowledge there are benefits for seniors consuming Cannabis. In all the years working with seniors I've witnessed many instances of over-medicating seniors, interactions with different medicines, or intolerance of medicines. Many of these medicines prescribed to the elderly slow down digestion and bowel function which causes constipation. This induces other serious health conditions for seniors whereas substituting Cannabis reduces occurrences of many reported side effects and health risks.

Introducing medicinal Cannabis is becoming more of an option, at least in San Diego, where I talked with my dad's neurosurgeon about Cannabis for my dad's pain management. The doctor told my dad, "We are going to have an intelligent conversation about Cannabis, Mr. Mitchell, and we are going with your daughter's plan for you." For an older surgeon to be on board with me administering Cannabis to my dad to help alleviate his pain and anxiety is encouraging and shows that times are changing.

What are the misconceptions about Cannabis?

The biggest misconception has been classifying it as a Schedule 1 Drug with no medicinal properties. Research has proven this false. This halted all research and education on the endocannabinoid system and the Cannabis plant. Cannabis is referred to as the plant with 1001 molecules; scientists are discovering many cannabinoids in the plant, not just THC and CBD. Research is validating that Cannabis has medicinal properties.

Maybe it's due to the movies and TV shows, but Cannabis consumers have typically been portrayed as lazy, stoners, slackers, and stupid which is the furthest from the truth for myself and many Cannabis consumers. I lived at high altitude in a ski town in Colorado for almost 15 years. We were athletic year-round from snow sports to summer hiking; many of us consumed Cannabis regularly and were fit (exceptionally fit) and successful business owners.

What questions are you most frequently asked?

1. Will this help me?
2. Will I overdose?
3. Will I get addicted?
4. Can I take it with all my meds?
5. Is Cannabis legal to consume if you reside in senior living communities?

The quick answer to many of these questions is yes, Cannabis can help most people with few side effects and without causing addiction or overdose deaths. Many medical professionals and scientists agree that Cannabis and CBD have a fairly good safety profile with limited drug interactions and side effects.

It serves no purpose when seniors take too much Cannabis as it might scare them from using it again. While there is no risk of overdose death, a person can overdose or rather over-consume and feel high or intoxicated. This makes them uncomfortable; too stressed and unbalanced. Cannabis and CBD can lower blood pressure, so again, if you use Cannabis medicinally, consult with your medical doctors.

Lastly, until Cannabis is legalized nationwide, I recommend older adults that reside in senior living communities check with their family, financial, and legal teams to ensure a safe and legal way to consume Cannabis without the risk of being evicted. Things are changing and more Cannabis educational events are happening for senior communities, but until it's fully legal, know your rights and how to consume legally so you don't jeopardize your living situation.

What questions should seniors and their loved ones ask?

1. How did you get your parents to finally use Cannabis and CBD?
2. Does it provide better sleep?
3. Can I relax without being intoxicated or high?
4. Will I have a higher risk of falling after using CBD and Cannabis?

For adult children that want their parents to use Cannabis, or at least consider it, they must realize that it's going to require many conversations with your senior loved ones. Take the time to really talk about modern Cannabis in context to the science and technology of modern Cannabis and relate it to any cultural issues. Many communities have had generations of family members incarcerated for Cannabis offenses, so now it's hard to see Cannabis as a medicine and a good thing. We must continue the dialogue to help communities grow into Cannabis acceptance.

Poor sleep is one of the top complaints from seniors. The Centers for Disease Control (CDC) reports that adults sleeping less than seven hours a night are more likely to report the top 10 chronic health conditions as compared to people that got enough sleep. Some of these top 10 health conditions affected by sleep disorders and lack of regular sleep include coronary heart disease, depression, and heart attacks. Lack of sleep throws off an individual's circadian rhythm, which is our innate biological feature that is basically our internal 24-hour clock that regulates many systems in our bodies. Lack of sleep can cause major disruption in our sleep-wake cycle which is all related to sleep patterns and health conditions. All of this negatively affects seniors that have a consistent lack of sleep.

A well-known San Diego cardiologist recently reached out to me to discuss sleep, seniors, and Cannabis. He told me it's the number one reason his senior patients are now asking him about Cannabis use. We continue to discuss Cannabis and he's researching it and talking with my clients that are his patients.

Seniors using Cannabis as a sleep aid is great as long as the senior understands that while you won't die from overdosing or overconsumption, you can get very sleepy/groggy or have a "high"/intoxicating feeling from using too much Cannabis. Since seniors get up often in the middle of the night to use the restroom, it's important to ensure they don't over-consume Cannabis and create a high risk for falls or other injuries. Remember, balance can be an issue for many, so regulating Cannabis consumption throughout the day is important for fall prevention measures.

Give me a few examples of a positive experience, benefits, or success stories.

Cannabis is part of my story and has contributed to the success of my life. I was able to get through trauma and thrive. This medicinal plant has been helping me with anxiety and pain management for most of my life. I have used it for menstruation cramping and accompanying nausea and now use it for managing menopause symptoms. When I was a high-altitude athlete, I regularly used Cannabis for muscle recovery and pain management. My mother started consuming Cannabis last year and we

166 · VERONICA MITCHELL

are monitoring it closely. I'm writing a series about my parents and their use of Cannabis for the first time in their lives. My mother's bowel and gut issues have been improving drastically and we are hopeful she will continue to improve. My dad's anxiety associated with his upcoming hip replacement surgery is being managed with Cannabis.

One of my clients was unsure how to initiate a Cannabis conversation with her entire family and her mother's doctors, so I worked with a local family and long-distance family members to have regular educational discussions with their mother and her medical team. The family reports their mother says she is sleeping better and most of the family is now supporting their matriarch using Cannabis.

With any new health practice, routine, or medicinal supplements, always start by consulting the entire healthcare and medical team. This is especially true for seniors as many have compromised immune systems, age-related illnesses, and take multiple prescriptions. So before introducing Cannabis, be sure that it's safe and all medical professionals are aware. Most Cannabis medical professionals recommend starting slow and low or "micro-dosing" Cannabis which means starting with a very small quantity of Cannabis, like .5 mg, and gradually increasing dosage amount while monitoring all effects of the Cannabis to find the right dose for each individual.

Depending on what your treating, many advise to layer your Cannabis intake, or use an entourage effect which means using several types of delivery systems from inhaling or smoking Cannabis, using a topical cream, ingesting a tincture and sublingual tablet, or eating an edible. Choosing the delivery system that works for an individual is a personal decision for every Cannabis user. The good thing is with all the new science and technology of the legal Cannabis industry, most people will find a delivery system that works best for them. The Arthritis

Foundation recently released CBD guidelines which are also proof that Cannabis acceptance is happening in America.

Senior living communities will eventually have to accept Cannabis and CBD consumption by their residents. With more medical professionals recommending Cannabis consumption and it is becoming legal throughout the nation, seniors and their families will demand access to it where they live. Regulations and safety protocols will be introduced to manage senior Cannabis consumption.

Until there is full legalization of Cannabis, meaning that it's legal in all states, consumers need to know their local laws and the laws where they purchase and travel with their CBD. Consumers should not risk penalty or criminal citations for Cannabis. Know your laws and how to consume Cannabis legally.

It is important that you purchase CBD or Cannabis from a legal dispensary or source. Legal compliant CBD and Cannabis are lab-tested and have been vetted to ensure it is safe for consumption. Do your due diligence and verify products and brands before spending money. Safeguard your health and wealth.

Are there any questions that you feel you would like to address that were not asked?

Seniors need education about and real-life experience with Cannabis to be able to make good decisions. I advise seniors that simply attending Cannabis events, getting on a bus to visit a dispensary and talk to vendors is not always the best avenue to finding the right products that work with their biochemistry and health conditions. Teaching new Cannabis users to understand that budtenders and retail staff at dispensaries are there to sell the products they need to sell to make a profit.

With that being said, you can find great dispensaries and wonderful teams inside those dispensaries that do have knowledge and education on working with seniors. I advise everyone to find places to purchase their Cannabis products that are trusted, reliable, legal, and compliant.

Buyer Beware

That adage is true: buyer beware. With the green rush of legal Cannabis and CBD comes many scam products and people scamming buyers. With CBD and Cannabis seemingly being sold everywhere, it can make it difficult for seniors to know what are real and quality products. It's imperative that canna-consumers purchase only from legal dispensaries and sources. Many seniors are living on a fixed income and Cannabis is very cost-prohibitive. It's not covered under insurance and the taxes are tremendous. Canna-seniors must ensure they get what they pay for and the ingredients are safe. Many claims are being made about products and ingredients without any substantiated proof or evidence of benefits. Some products contain so little Cannabis and CBD that it's not measurable, making it "snake oil," with no medicinal properties.

Go with your seniors to Cannabis events and protect them from giving out personal information or consuming unsafe products. Verify all brands and products before seniors start consuming. Make it a point to assist them create and design their canna-wellness lifestyle. Be a part of their Cannabis exploration and help your senior loved one find the right CBD and Cannabis products that work for them in the correct dosages.

It's never too late for seniors to start consideration of this plant medicine. Help them learn and be a part of it for them and yourself.

Veronica Mitchell

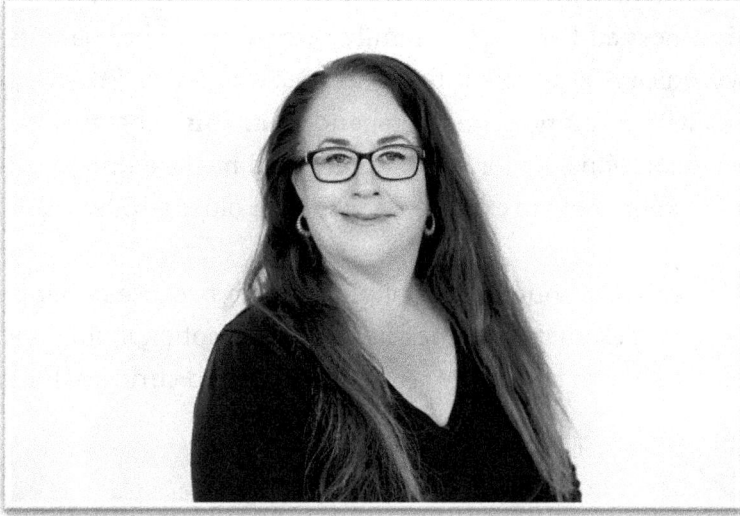

Veronica Mitchell is a writer, consultant, and speaker based in San Diego, CA. She was the founder of two successful corporations in Vail, CO and San Diego, CA. She has a passion for business, advocating for women and seniors, and she is a caregiver for her parents. Veronica is a survivor of childhood sexual abuse. She navigates her trauma survival into trauma growth with resilience, mental and physical healthcare, and Cannabis. She has used Cannabis as part of her plant medicine for many years. She incorporates years of practicing Eastern and alternative medicine with Western medicine to create a balanced approach for her healthcare for the mind and body.

Born in Brooklyn, NY, her father worked for the Federal Government and they lived in Memphis, TN, before her dad got transferred to Washington, DC where she spent her formidable years growing up in Montgomery County, MD. She attended Montgomery College in Rockville, MD, until she decided to spend one ski season in Vail, CO. She did not return to the East Coast to live and built a life and business in the Vail Valley. She is an outdoorswoman and thoroughly enjoyed living in the Rocky Mountains. She helped her sister start a transportation and caregiving business in San Diego where she eventually moved to join the business and assist with family caregiving for her parents.

Veronica is now consulting and speaking around the United States with **Seniors, Caregivers, and Cannabis**™ because families, corporations, senior communities, and medical professionals want to know how to explore Cannabis for older adults and caregivers.

Veronica is a sought-after public speaker because of her genuine approach that combines her verbal, emotional, and social intelligence with her funny sense of humor and curiosity for life.

AC Moon

Reinvention of a State of Mind

I turned over in my bed, snuggling with the softness of my handstitched baby blanket, listening to the moans of my hard-working mother's pain erupt from her as she found herself finally at rest for the day. As always, I felt her pain.

Life's habit was that the morning came early, and I ate my granola as I watched her crippled hands unscrew the dozens of bottles of medications, compiling them one at a time in front of her in rows. Grabbing each tiny colored pill and gulping it down with a mouthful of coffee.

This tradition of cancer, arthritis, lupus, Graves' disease pharmaceutical morning cocktails was nonstop. Some of my earliest childhood memories were of my physically tortured mother telling me that she must take these handfuls of pills or she will go to sleep and never wake up. As a kid, I tried to help her with mud pies and food colored toast to no avail, and so I vowed at an early age that I would find a way to help her with the pain.

Later in life, it developed into an outright disgust with "Big Pharma."

Mom taught me the ways of self-sustaining homestead life and the many ways of using the land and plants around us to survive and heal ourselves. Yet the teachings of Cannabis were taboo in her generation, brainwashed into a social reefer madness that no one really understood. Being as she raised me in very remote areas of mountains, I quickly realized that I was surrounded endlessly with herbal knowledge and began my training in medical "marijuana" at age 13. The many years of childhood gardening sowed the seeds for a lifetime of dedication to medical Cannabis.

Years later, I sat cross legged amidst groups of aging tie-dyed souls. Gathered 'round huge fields of organic Cannabis we tended to so meticulously. There was a gamut of ailments within the community and each person used every aspect of the plant in some form to create a healing element within their lives. We supplied our collective dispensaries with "medical marijuana" in order to help patients, feed the gardens, and ourselves. That midday, we tuned in on the radio as we worked, and through those waves we hear the glorious outcry from the D.J., "California HAS JUST PASSED THE BILL FOR MEDICAL MARIJUANA!" We all stood up and cheered for all the warriors before us that paved the way to what we thought was our new freedom. "Cannabis cures cancer!" we chanted! "Down with Big Pharma!"

But I was only 16 and that was just the beginning of legalizing medical Cannabis. As of last year, California is now a LEGAL Cannabis state. Anyone over the age of 18 can consume it privately. And, I am now over twice that age. It has taken almost my entire life to see the legalization of Cannabis and the household use of elements such as CBD. Unfortunately, on a state level, the laws passed were not in favor of patients' rights, but the healers continue onward, each in their own ways, and CBD in hemp form has become available to the public nationwide. Medical focus has continued to be driven by the organic pioneers that believe in its healing abilities as well as entrepreneurs from every walk of life.

This revolutionary state, as well as many others, have set steppingstones for our ability to cultivate, compile, derive, concentrate, and educate ourselves on over 120 different type of phytocannibinoids.

THC (tetrahydrocannabinol) and CBD. (cannabidiol) are two of the most well-known of the cannabinoids. These elements provide "anti-inflammatory" or "intoxicating" attributes. THC, known to get a person "high" or provide direct pain relief, and CBD, being of "antioxidant and anti-inflammatory" effect. Many others, including CBG and CBC play roles in creating different combinations of effects and it is important to understand the plant source you have available to you as well as any allergies you may have.

Each one of the many phytocannabinoids has a unique and important link in the mystical code of our personal cannabinoid receptor systems. Some people may have some receptors blocked due to diet or genetics while others may have an extreme sensitivity. These factors can all play a role in how things mesh with you. It is up to the patient to determine what is right for them. This keeps the true medical freedom within your ability to experiment with real results and feel for yourself the difference a plant can make in your life.

Take the time to read labels or ask questions and research. When in doubt, always grab organic. When cooking with or learning to work with the plant extracts, please test as you go in small quantities, to allow yourself to learn from your experiences and improve them. As a consumer of lotions, topicals, edibles, concentrates, etc., educate yourself on the delivery systems and what's inside your new products. This new era of obtainability has given room to a lot of "snake oils" and toxic uncertified corner store yuck.

I personally advocate for growing your own plant and being a part of the amazing cycle of what is herbal medicines. There are many resources available on obtaining legal hemp seeds or Cannabis seeds and education on how to do it yourself and I will share some little easy treasures of DYI further on in the chapter.

In 2001, I started my first medical marijuana edibles and cultivation collective. Harvest Moon Munchie Company. Made up of over 160 doctor-certified patients of all forms. My mission was to provide the highest quality homegrown product to as many patients as possible at the very lowest price. I often dedicated endless days and nights making free infused candies and goodies of all forms to give the poverty ridden cancer and AIDS patients of the Bay. Later, southern California became the gateway for strong movement in the medical marijuana sector and we provided dozens of collectives, organic infusions, and flower to curb the destitute from opiate addictions. Cannabis in all forms is a must for the recovery of many mortal chemical addicts and is at a current pivot point of social discussions on how to implement it into recovery centers.

One evening I was closing the dispensary with some friends and a lady 'round sixty years old came to the counter, caught my attention, and told me a story, " Last night, I had some of your 'Bomb-Bomb'(truffles) candies in the refrigerator on a plate to chill. I have a mostly bed-ridden mother, whom rarely goes out of her room; she's almost ninety years old. Last night apparently, she discovered your candies and ate one. She has not really spoken or walked around much in years. I was really worried when I found out but, late last night I want you to know I had the longest conversation with my mother I have in a decade... your candy brought my mom back to me!" The woman started toward me and gave me a huge hug with tears in her eyes, and I knew that no matter what happened, I couldn't give up on this path I was on. I spoke with the woman many times through the months as she learned to use Cannabis to navigate the pains of life and her ailing mother. I'll never forget that woman. We changed each other forever.

Through decades of professional cultivation and college educations, certifications, and so on, I now professionally consult on everything from phenotypes to infusions and new product innovations. I began my consulting team, Indica Innovations International, where we bring medical "marijuana" and CBD Hemp integration into new medically legal nations. Consulting internationally on medical Cannabis has given me a broad perspective of how this one plant can change the life of an entire country, one patient at a time. It is widely known that hemp can singularly save the planet. The Cannabis plant that doesn't get you "high" (less than .3% THC) and provides our long sought out CBD compound. Not only does this plant provide more resources and textiles than any other plant on the globe, it also has amazing medical properties, health benefits, and is the missing link in many humans' diets. Not to mention it provides an exceptional amount of oxygen to the atmosphere.

CBD can be found in a handful of known botanical entities on the planet. One of them being a white pine tree as well as two types of mint. The element is commonly extracted from large droves of hemp plants. Full spectrum extract implies that the entire biomass was used to extract present elements while hemp oil is often cold pressed from seeds. These, I focus on being health benefits, such as an abundance of omegas and fatty acids which have multiple sustained nutrients to go so far as boosting metabolism and reducing aging.

CBD concentrated oils can be found at dispensaries and other locations made from the traditional Cannabis hybrid flowers that have been medically bred to provide low THC high CBD tests. This choice is often the finest quality with the most proficient and expedited effect. Though it may have trace amounts of THC, unlike those derived from hemp plants (Cannabis ruderalis), it does not alter mindset. I have seen evidence that the partnering of said cannabinoids with proper diet can cure cancer. Rick Simpson oil or "Phoenix Tears" is an isolate recipe of 1:1 ratio using alcohol to naturally distill the elements into a medical tincture. I believe in this recipe if made correctly and you can research it fully online to see the tear-jerking stories yourself. Again, be aware and read labels thoroughly before use as well as allow for personal testing of the products to get to know the herb. Thankfully, unlike all those nasty pill side effects, the worst side effect you could get from experimenting with Cannabis CBD is a good night's rest.

You want your labels to show you the origin of the CBD. Is it full spectrum, hemp oil or CBD flower derived? Is it organic? Is there THC present and if so, how much? Is it from a reliable source? Is it from the United States? Other countries have much different standards and a large abundance of hemp derivatives are being imported from Asia where toxic growing practices are used. Know your source. Better yet, know your grower. And, even better than that, become your own herbal gardener.

You can each try growing your own little hemp or Cannabis plant at home. Depending on your state for Cannabis that is, but for hemp, it's totally safe and legal. Research hemp seeds for sale and make sure, again, it's from a reputable source such as those recommended by Grow Magazine and Hemp Associates of America. It's easy to germinate a seed like a flower and give it a bit of fertilizer. If it gets too tall just go ahead and cut it shorter until the time of year when it starts throwing out small flowering hairs (pistols). It will take about 9 weeks for it to fully mature into bloom. At that point, you will have little CBD flowers at no cost, right in your own home. It's easy to dry. When flowers have fully bloomed, and you see the hairs upon the blossoms turn amber, go ahead and cut it down and hang it in the shed to dry until crisp.

An easy, quick CBD oil recipe is taking the hemp flower and grinding it up into a low cooking organic coconut oil. Let it cook for few hours then strain it with cheese cloth and, voilà; you can cook with it, adding your own CBD to every recipe or have it on hand for a great infused coconut rub and topical ointment for aches and pains. My mother, who was against the smoking of Cannabis, found huge relief from arthritis and lupus from my homemade topicals. You can also do this with isolates and store-bought CBD oils for creative healthy ideas. There's pretty much nothing you can't do with CBD and Cannabis. Be prepared in the near future to have it added as optional into anything in creation. Think of your goal on using Cannabis or CBD. Are you healing?

Looking for preventative health benefits? Pain relief? Curious on Cannabis culture? Once you know what type of "end result" you are looking for in this plant, the much easier it will be to obtain it.

My love for plants, combined with a passion for creativity and homestead ways, I had always found myself at times in positions of need (especially when those storms start rolling in). I have always loved the protective and controllable feel of greenhouse cultivating and have always strived and thrived with home growers while teaching what a little bit of assistance can do for the botanical entities. Especially when living in high elevation or unrestful climates where any type of plant is at risk for the punishments of weather or pests.

All this organic love brought about my first federally patented invention, Croptops Greenhouses. Too many years of fighting with Mother Nature, she wanted me to find a way to be harmonious in my growing with her. "Croptops" is an instant portable greenhouse that protects plants of all forms from storms. Furthermore, it found great feedback being used for quarantine for pest control and isolation areas for cloning, tissue culture, and so on. The journey of becoming an inventor has been arduous, and I continue it presently, hoping to make a difference every day that I possibly can. I look forward to being able to take my entrepreneurial ideas each to the next level. There isn't a day that goes by where I don't have another idea. I encourage each of you reading to live in the creative space of your mind and the lucid space of your body, create, invent, innovate, and thrive!

Now is the time to revolutionize the world with our commitment to transparent science-based knowledge. Use the internet and homegrown resources to learn past the ever-daunting stigma of Cannabis use. CBD is a zillion dollar industry worldwide and as the people of the planet begin to understand the multitude of positive aspects that can come from hemp and Cannabis, we gain power as a species.

Almost all things once started out as plants. We demonize some, yet others sustain value. A poppy once grown for a toothache and surgery in eastern Asia now spreads the globe toxifying bodies in the form of chemically treated "heroine." Yet we need it medically for morphine. Cannabis and hemp are not the type of plants that cause that effect in any form. But this is another example on how society abused a plant into toxicity. Alcohol was once even considered a medical aid; now an astringent. "Cocaine," (coca plant) used for Novocain - another abused plant. Even the bark of a type of birch tree is now just common "Aspirin." They remove the name of the plant and synthesize it in order to gain control over its assets and exploit it. Centuries of plant knowledge has been lost in capitalizing on the natures of the species. That is why it is so important for us all to continue seeking and gaining knowledge; experimenting and innovating new ways of looking at these ancient things we call, plants.

Cannabis Heals and is safe to use in many ways.

CBD does not cause most people to feel high if it is hemp derived. Hemp has zero THC (euphoric effect).

No matter what we do, there is no "miracle plant", as we wished for. Though Cannabis is pretty close to magic, as is aloe and so many others, we must remain conscious of all aspects of our existence. Be aware how you carry yourself and your posture. Eat healthy and unprocessed foods as much as possible; carry organic thoughts and make it a priority to take yourself to a garden and sit with nature as much as possible.

And remember; to grow as a person - that is truly the recipe for getting high on Life.

Healing the mind, body, and soul,

AC Moon

About AC Moon

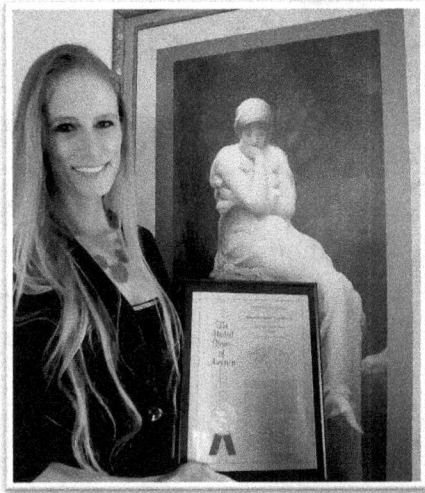

Diverse Certified Master Grower with more than 20 years of Cannabis experience. Ms. Moon is dedicated to the art of innovation and integration within the Horticultural Cannabis Industry.

After an off-grid childhood in the gardens of Northern California, AC Moon launched Harvest Moon Munchie Co. in 2001. One of the first non-chlorophyll concentrate based medical edibles companies in the area. Partnered with brokering and educating the populace on the benefits of organic herbal remedies, AC later diversified and continues to provide high quality infusions, education, and genetics throughout many areas within the state and beyond.

Encompassing different locations and properties, she used her skills to purchase, develop, and grow substantial amounts of high-quality cannabinoids in several ecosystems and climates, ensuring the success of each plantation from propagation to fruition while managing multiple agricultural teams in remote locations. Simultaneously, she used her college obtained environmental horticultural knowledge to remediate prior land damage and reoccur organic structure within local ecosystems, as well as teach "best practices" and "light deprivation" techniques in those locations. She also partook in various partnerships with Medical Cannabis dispensaries and cooperatives for distribution.

While gathering research through the years within many aspects of "the plant", AC Moon began taking her product innovations to the next level. Her first patent (granted in 2018 with 21 micro patents) was Croptops Greenhouses of Croptopsgreenhouses.com. "Instant Portable Greenhouse." She continues to seek partnerships for her plethora of intellectual properties and consults on various stages of cultivating, product innovations, intellectual property management, trademarking, and business creation.

AC also attended school for product and licensing in the mainstream world. She later began writing online college courses to teach her hard earned education to other struggling entrepreneurs.

In the future, she hopes to create a certifiable process for clean, green, productive growing within commercial growing recreational operations on a large level as well as innovate products to help ensure successes.

Private clients in the product development of both cultivating and intellectual property have also enlisted her services to develop strategies for research and development of their organically used products in the Cannabis world. She continues to strengthen and build relationships in the culture within media and business connections as the new industry develops into mainstream.

Ms. Moon has a well-known, refutable reputation in the Cannabis industry and is continuing to write for columns and magazines to spread the words of our culturally indicative community into business platforms. Supported by various business owners, inventors, and home growers, AC relishes in the opportunities to interact with many integrated aspects of the industry and use her creative skills to facilitate uprising businesses globally into their primes.

MEDICAL

Thelma Cela

Tell me about your journey with Cannabis and your area of expertise.

As VP of Clinical Operations for OrthoNOW, I review the quality improvement of our clinical programs as well as new care models and their effectiveness.

OrthoNOW operates a network of orthopedic care clinics in south Florida that deliver on-demand care for all musculoskeletal injuries and pain. Our clinics have treated over 14,000 cases of which the largest percentage of conditions involve patients experiencing pain and/or inflammation. Traditionally, OrthoNOW clinicians would prescribe a variety of non-steroidal anti-inflammatory (NSAIDS) or recommend an analgesic for the pain.

In years past, there were cases which warranted a stronger course of prescription medication and the clinician would prescribe a narcotic to relieve the pain. Like many other healthcare providers, OrthoNOW became very concerned with the increase of opioid addiction in our country and in south Florida, and we instituted protocols to manage pain without the use of narcotics or opioids. The orthopedic care clinics have been diligently putting measures in place in order to become an "opioid free" healthcare facility.

Traditional physical therapy is a modality used to address the management of pain for patients. In addition to traditional physical therapy, the company was exploring pain management options including incorporating electro neuromuscular therapy as part of the rehabilitation services OrthoNOW provides our patients. With the use of an electric stimulator that can work in different frequencies to recruit either slow-twitch muscle fibers (stability muscles) or fast-twitch muscle fibers (strength and power muscles), we can relax those guarded muscles and improve blood flow rich in nutrients.

The developed protocols and diagnosis techniques can first assess the area of injury where the kinetic chain is causing the poor movement and is the origin of injury rather than the damaged tissue. By reducing edema and muscle guarding first, we are putting the body in the optimum environment for healing, accelerating the recovery process while re-educating the "NEURO-MUSCULAR" connection to address the origin of the injury, and restoring proper mechanics which leads in long-term prevention of injuries.

We also began offering patients relief from pain and inflammation with plasma rich protein (PRP) therapy as another treatment option. Packed with growth and healing factors, platelets initiate repair and attract the critical assistance of stem cells. Platelet rich plasma therapy's natural healing process intensifies the body's efforts by delivering a higher concentration of platelets. A small sample of the patient's blood is drawn (similar to a lab test sample) and placed in a centrifuge that spins the blood at high speeds, separating the platelets from the other components. The concentrated PRP injection is then delivered into and around the point of injury, jump-starting and significantly strengthening the body's natural healing signal. Because the patient's own blood is used (it is autologous), there is no risk of a transmissible infection and a very low risk of allergic reaction.

For very complex orthopedic issues, OrthoNOW has given mesenchymal stem cell injections. These are used occasionally for those conditions that require diverse cell migration and differentiation to assist in the healing process such as a long bone non-union or deficient wound bed for healing.

Like the therapies mentioned before, we continued to maintain an interest in searching for alternatives to medications, injections, and rehabilitation therapy. This approach to embracing new and innovative technologies is what led us to exploring the benefits that CBD therapy could offer our patient population.

When did your interest start in Cannabis and why?

OrthoNOW's interest began through communications with colleagues and professional associates. OrthoNOW was able to learn about the use of CBD or "cannabidiol" for pain management and as an anti-inflammatory and started our journey into having CBD as a therapy for our patients' pain management and inflammation reduction.

CBD is one of more than 100 identified molecules in the hemp and Cannabis or marijuana plant. We learned that CBD is non-psychoactive. Every part of us – from our brain to our internal organs to our respiratory and muscular systems – has what are called CBD receptors. CBD stimulates the endocannabinoid system (ECS) which researchers have linked to many processes such as chronic pain, stress, inflammation, mood, sleep, cardiovascular system, and many others. These functions all contribute to homeostasis, or your body's internal environment's stability. Experts believe that maintaining homeostasis is the primary role of the ECS and that CBD works by preventing the endocannabinoids from being broken down. This allows them to have more of an effect on the body. Others believe that CBD binds to a receptor.

As OrthoNOW continued to learn more and more about CBD and its benefits, the company knew we had to research suppliers to identify those whose products were aligned with the medical grade product we needed to have associated with our brand.

We found such a company to partner with and were able to successfully launch a line of CBD products under the name of *OrthoNaturals*. The CBD product line include:

- <u>OrthoNaturals CBD 300 mg Lotion</u> - which is good for localized pain and can last up to five (5) hours. This product can also be used for skin rehydration, psoriasis, and dermatitis.

- <u>OrthoNaturals CBD 300 mg Muscle Cream</u> – this product is applied liberally to the tight or painful muscles. Also designed to be used as a massage cream, if desired.

- <u>OrthoNaturals CBD 750 mg Freeze Roll-On</u> - this is great for post workout or for relief from sore joints and muscles. This product is also for localized treatment and can last up to five (5) hours.

- <u>OrthoNaturals CBD 500 mg Tincture with Terpenes</u> - this is the fastest acting CBD product we have which patients report feeling the effect within 30 minutes and lasting anywhere from 2-4 hours after being taken. This is a sublingual product (which is placed beneath the tongue), held for about 30 seconds, and then swallowed. This is indicated for decreasing inflammation and reducing pain.

What are the misconceptions of Cannabis?

One of the misconceptions of CBD is that it is THC, or tetra-hydrocannabinol. People think if you use a product containing CBD, you will get the same effects that you would if you consume something with THC or marijuana. THC is one of the main can-nabinoids found in Cannabis. It is the psychoactive compound that gets you "high." These psychoactive properties are part of the side effects of THC which include memory loss, dry mouth, increased heart rate, coordination problems, and red eyes. CBD is well tolerated, even in large quantities; however, if THC is used in high amounts, it may be connected to some long-term negative psychiatric effects.

Another misconception of CBD is that it is illegal to purchase. Patients sometimes ask whether they might even get arrested for purchasing CBD products. In December 2018, the federal government passed the Federal Farm Bill 2018 legalizing hemp CBD. The Farm Bill ensures that any cannabinoid—a set of chemical compounds found in the Cannabis plant—that is derived from hemp will be legal, if and only if that hemp is produced in a manner consistent with the Farm Bill, associated federal regulations, association state regulations, and by a licensed grower. CBD derived from hemp is legal in Florida and in all 50 states.

What questions are you most frequently asked?

(1) Because OrthoNOW is a healthcare clinic, a common question a patient will ask is whether the CBD product being recommended is going to be reimbursed by their health plan. Currently, there is no formulary coverage for any CBD-based prescription alternative but, OrthoNOW set the pricing for the CBD products to be comparable to Medicare and most commercial insurance co-pays or deductibles making access to the products desirable by the patient.

Pricing the products we sell at OrthoNOW was a challenge as well. Because of the hype for all CBD products in the market, there is a myriad of things being sold. The items we have at our clinics are competitively priced, but for some consumers, the price points might seem high. Our staff were trained by our vendor partner on the features and benefits of the products. As we continue to offer this pain relief option, we will continue to monitor literature and product information to remain vigilant of any industry changes or additions. We will continue to tell our patients that at no point can we guarantee that a false positive on a drug test will not occur. CBD and THC at this point are difficult to distinguish in field tests and other quantifiable drug tests. We do not recommend you take the product if this is a sensitive issue at your workplace. We also encourage the patients to have a conversation with their employer or with the workers compensation adjuster and show them the third-party reports for all CBD products OrthoNOW carries to initiate a conversation.

(2) An OrthoNOW patient might inquire, particularly many of our workers compensation patients, whether this product can be detected in a drug screen test or toxicology panel. We treat many officers and military personnel and they are routinely tested randomly so they too will be very interested in knowing whether this product is detected in drug panels. There is 0.0% of THC in any of the products offered to patients at OrthoNOW. This concern is a natural one on the part of these patients as any levels of THC in their system will be considered a drug test failure and could jeopardize their workers compensation claims. THC would result in a "positive" drug test.

Our therapists and clinicians are very careful to share that we are in the initial stages of this CBD boom and as such, we simply cannot be 100% sure of any claims made by manufacturers or suppliers. OrthoNOW will maintain a cautious position with this patient population and make sure to educate them on the very slim chance that a random drug test might report a positive result derived from using a CBD product. As a company, we feel it is safest and most appropriate to err on the side of caution until we have regulation and governmental oversight on all these products.

(3) Another question OrthoNOW is asked is regarding the effectiveness of one CBD product versus another in the line we offer our patients. Every staff member at our OrthoNOW clinics has been educated on the different forms of delivery and rates of

absorption for our CBD products. The products OrthoNOW has available range from tinctures, which have the fastest absorption rate, typically within 30 minutes, and lasts for about 2-4 hours, to topicals which are good for localized treatment but could last up to 5 hours.

(4) Patients also ask if CBD has any drug interactions. CBD can affect the body like grapefruit and inhibits the cytochrome P450 system. CBD can reduce or increase the effects of certain prescribed medications by interacting with receptors throughout the body's endocannabinoid system (ECS) and by inhibiting the activity of cytochrome P450. Cytochrome P450 is a group of liver enzymes that are responsible for breaking down drugs and toxins that enter the body. By inhibiting the activity of this enzyme, CBD can temporarily deactivate its activity, which can alter how other compounds are metabolized. The medications to be most concerned about are blood thinners like Coumadin. By slowing down how the body metabolizes these drugs, CBD preserves the medication's durability and prolongs its presence in the body. Effectively, CBD can increase and prolong the effects of drugs that increase the risk of bleeding, and the usage of both simultaneously should be closely monitored by a medical professional. OrthoNOW tells our patients who take blood thinners to tell their prescribing physician that you are on CBD and he or she might want to check your blood levels more frequently than they usually do.

What questions should people be asking?

Consumers should be asking what exactly is found in the CBD product they are considering taking. Because of the recent explosion in the market that CBD products have had and the interest level on the part of the consumer, many savvy retailers and entrepreneurs have jumped on the CBD bandwagon and are offering products. OrthoNOW recommends the buyer look carefully at the product label. Read the ingredients to look for CBD in the list. There are products being sold with a CBD name but contain a mix of oil and menthol and are being touted as a "great CBD pain relief product." Look for things like organic hemp seed oil, myrcene terpene or CBD + myrcene. Also, look for things like hemp-derived cannabidiol (CBD).

The consumer should also look for a CBD product which has been tested by an independent third-party company and that the certificate of this testing is provided to the consumer to review.

OrthoNOW's products all have a QR code on the bottle which links to the company website with each batch's certificate of laboratory testing results.

Give an example of a positive experience with or benefits of cannabidiol (CBD).

The CBD products OrthoNOW carries have demonstrated benefits as an antipsychotic, antidepressant, anti-inflammatory, antioxidant, neuroprotective, appetite control, analgesic for rheumatoid arthritis, anti-ischemic (prevents plaque build-up in arteries), and anti-emetic. OrthoNaturals' CBD products are an all-natural solution to our body's aches and pains.

Give an example of how CBD has been life changing for someone you know.

We cannot say that the CBD products we offer our patients are "life changing" as that is a relative concept. What we can report is that by having this natural alternative to pain management and inflammation relief, our patients say they are grateful to have this option available. There are many patients who prefer alternatives to traditional medicines. There are others who simply choose not to take anything requiring prescriptions and would prefer a product without any medicinal component in it.

OrthoNOW is pleased to have found products free from medicines but are still effective in minimizing or eliminating pain and discomfort.

What changes in the industry do you see coming in the future?

We don't have enough experience in this "industry" yet to make a fair statement here. It is new to us, but it is exciting to be part of a growing industry.

What do you wish people knew or understood about Cannabis?

We want the average consumer to take the time to educate themselves about ALL of the alternatives to traditional medicines which are available to them, including Cannabis, or CBD. People create assumptions based on outdated or incorrect information and in this CBD industry, there exists many false or outdated beliefs. Many stem from the association to marijuana or THC. If we mention "Cannabis," the knee-jerk reaction is to think about a person getting high on a marijuana joint. Perhaps books like this one where facts are being presented about CBD is a great start. Educating the public on CBD will go a long way toward helping many who might find relief from pain or benefit from one of its many other applications.

OrthoNOW provider patient stories

As OrthoNOW operates orthopedic specialty walk-in care clinics, you would expect that the majority, if not all, of the patients seen experience pain to varying degrees. In fact, our data analytics demonstrate that of the top ten presenting diagnosis at OrthoNOW, 90% of them are PAIN – knee pain, back pain, neck pain, etc.

One of our providers interviewed for this chapter explained that along with his patients experiencing a certain level of pain associated with whatever their condition might be, they also are having trouble sleeping at night due to their pain. He has found that educating his patients about the additional benefits achieved from using a CBD product, like with the tinctures we recommend to our patients providing a restful night's sleep, becomes a deciding factor in whether a patient might try the product or not. Patients comment during their follow-up visits that the CBD product relaxed them, in addition to relieving their pain, and they feel like they finally got, "a good night's sleep." They also report to the provider that they do not feel any lingering effects when they wake up the next morning. They share that other prescription and non-prescription products they had tried resulted in having a groggy feeling upon waking up the next morning. This anecdotal account is then shared with other OrthoNOW clinicians so they can share with their patients as they discuss the features and benefits of CBD in pain management.

Another OrthoNOW clinician says that her patients, especially the older population, were the ones broaching the subject of CBD products for the pain and inflammation that brought them to our clinics. The provider had already started researching (on her own) about the efficacy of CBD, and then learned that OrthoNOW was looking at offering some products for sale at our centers. In this provider's experience, what she sees most from the patients is that they question the difference between the products OrthoNOW has available and what they see being sold at retail stores and even at gas stations. After some research online, we found that many of the "gas station CBD" oils being sold over the counter aren't CBD at all, instead containing other oils or potentially harmful substitutes.

OrthoNOW went through painstaking research and data collection when we were searching for a CBD supplier. Because we treat many workers compensation, military, police, and firefighters, we had to ensure the products we have available to ALL our patient population are free from THC and containing CBD.

This patient population is routinely drug tested. Any amount of THC would appear in the toxicity report. The vendor we chose and the products we identified to sell out of our clinics contain 0.0% THC. The milligrams of CBD vary by the type of product, but generally the range is from 250 mg of CBD to as much as 100 mg (in the products OrthoNOW carries). Our supplier partner has a large selection of products with much higher concentrations of CBD. Additionally, all of the products have hemp-derived CBD oil and 99% pure CBD isolate.

About Thelma Cela, FACHE, VP of Clinical Operations, OrthoNOW LLC

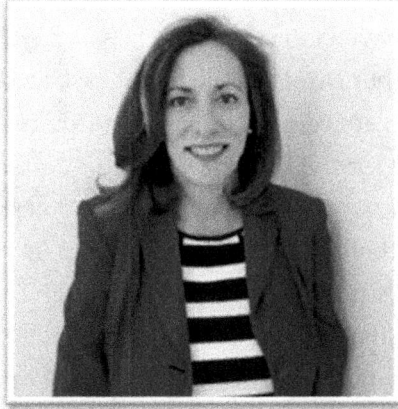

Since April 2016, Thelma Cela has served as Vice President of Clinical Operations for OrthoNOW®, the nation's only orthopedic walk-in care network of clinics. In this role, she provides day-to-day support on all clinical matters for all clinic locations. As Vice President of Clinical Operations, she sets direction on clinical policies and procedures and monitoring healthcare policy changes.

Before joining OrthoNOW®, Thelma had been recruited by Leon Medical Centers, a private healthcare company operating comprehensive medical centers to launch a new business line addressing the health and wellness of an aging population. As Director, Thelma researched and developed the company's Health Living Centers which provided first of its kind facilities in the south Florida market to offer services to the community of health aging.

Thelma has a proven track record in multiple corporate health-care cultures having worked for Mercy Hospital, where she was senior program director of their Diabetes Treatment Center and director of their surgical weight loss program. She enhanced the service line's awareness in the community, improved clinical outcomes for both illnesses, and built volume growth while maintaining ongoing physician support.

Thelma began her career in the healthcare arena after graduating from the University of Miami with a degree in psychology when she worked for the Epilepsy Foundation as their case manager. After a brief couple of months in the role, she assumed responsibility over their bi-weekly neurological clinic which served over 375,000 lives. She serves on the SSJ Health Foundation Board of Directors, has also served on the healthcare business council of the south Florida Hispanic Chamber of Commerce and is a graduate of the Greater Miami Leadership Class XV. Thelma will be graduating in May 2020, with a Master's degree in business administration with a concentration in healthcare and finance.

Thelma is Cuban born and immigrated to America at the age of two with her family. She has always lived in Miami, is married to Jose L. Cela, and they have a son, Brandon, who just graduated Cum Laude with a Bachelor of Arts degree in multi-media studies.

Justin Kander

Tell me about your journey with Cannabis and your area of expertise.

The use of Cannabis to treat cancer.

When did your interest in Cannabis start and why?

My primary interest was sparked in March 2008, when I saw the documentary *Run from the Cure* about a man named Rick Simpson administering high doses of THC-rich Cannabis extracts to terminal cancer patients and observing remissions. While there were many flaws with the documentary and Rick's approach, the key finding that sustained, high doses of cannabinoids could have an anticancer effect triggered significant interest in the medical Cannabis community and led to a dramatic accumulation of anecdotal evidence to accompany growing scientific evidence.

What are the misconceptions of Cannabis?

There are misconceptions on both sides. Some think Cannabis can do no harm, and others think Cannabis is far more dangerous than it really is. In regard to my field of interest, I think there is a strong misconception about the level of evidence showing how Cannabis fights cancer. Many believe there are only a few supporting studies and relatively weak anecdotal evidence. In reality, the evidence includes a double-blind, placebo-controlled trial, at least 100 documented cases and most likely thousands of anecdotal cases globally, and dozens of peer-reviewed studies showing how phytocannabinoids and endocannabinoids kill cancer cells through similar mechanisms.

What questions are you asked most frequently?

1. How much THC and CBD should be used for [form of cancer]?
2. What ratios of THC and CBD should be used for [form of cancer]?
3. What strains of Cannabis should be used for [form of cancer]?
4. What method of delivery should be used for [form of cancer]?
5. What are the success rates of Cannabis for treating [form of cancer]?

What questions should people be asking?

In addition to the frequently asked questions above, patients should have an understanding of how many milligrams of THC and CBD they are using/should be using, more importantly than measures of volume (milliliters or grams) or ratios (1:1, 1:4, etc.)

Give me a few examples of a positive experience, benefits, or success stories.

Cannabis extracts have been used to treat tumors for over 100 years and have seen many successes. In terms of Aunt Zelda's, we have had patients with terminal conditions who have gone into remission with Cannabis therapy, although there are no guarantees of such results for any individual patients. Outside Aunt Zelda's, many stories have been reported through various media outlets or videos. One particularly unique and surprising story concerned a man named Brian Stewart, an inductee of the Canadian Motorsports Hall of Fame, who used Cannabis oil to heal skin cancer in himself and two others.

https://cmhf.ca/brian-stewart/

https://www.youtube.com/watch?v=x8W1fIMxJE4

What are the recommended starting doses for animals? Can you overdose an animal and are there any side effects?

It is important to start animals with very low doses of either CBD or THC at 1 mg. CBD can likely be increased safely at 1-5 mg per day, but if THC is being used, it should be increased more slowly at .33-1 mg per day to avoid side effects. The same side effects that happen in humans can happen more extremely in animals if they overdose, including severe anxiety, nausea, vomiting, and convulsions. These usually happen when animals eat large quantities of THC. Using very small quantities of THC in a controlled manner appears safe in most cases.

Give me an example of how this was life changing for someone you know.

The first patient I ever worked with, Dennis Hill, used Cannabis therapy in conjunction with anti-hormone therapy to beat prostate cancer in 2011, which allowed him to avoid chemotherapy and radiation which had been suggested. He stayed healthy for years until getting lung cancer around 2018. At that point, he didn't want to use high doses of Cannabis again and used only small doses to deal with pain until passing in March 2019. He lived seemingly longer than expected with a conventionally untreated lung cancer and passed away very peacefully. Helping him initially beat cancer and making his last days so good, Cannabis was definitely life changing.

How has Cannabis helped you, clients, or others where other products were unsuccessful?

Cannabis has helped some people deal with all major symptom categories, such as pain, inflammation, anxiety, depression, and sleep where conventional medicines have failed.

What changes in the industry do you foresee coming in the future?

I foresee prices coming down dramatically, a consolidation of companies, and, most hopefully, the emergence of programs that provide Cannabis oil at steep discounts or free for cancer patients. That last part may take a while, but I believe it is inevitable.

What do you wish people knew or understood about Cannabis?

I wish people knew that it *really* can put terminal cancers into remission. It is clear that most in the industry don't understand that truth in their hearts or a revolution would have already come. There are still small vestiges of doubt, which is understandable, but I wish more people would take the time to see how strong the evidence is. People are dying because they don't have access to Cannabis medicine, and things will not change quickly without revolution.

What is important to look for when selecting a Cannabis product for a pet?

The same as for a person – a product that is completely absent of pesticides, molds, and heavy metals.

Justin Kander

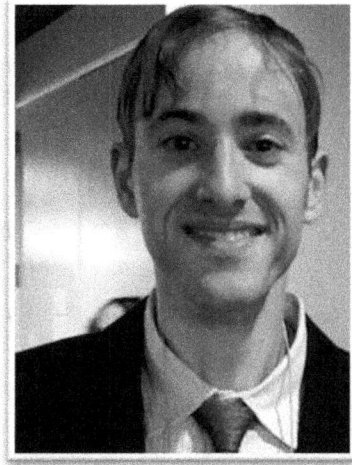

Justin Kander is the Research & Development Coordinator for The Oil Plant, a licensed California Cannabis manufacturer specializing in the production of Cannabis extracts, Cannabis-infused olive oils, and Cannabis topicals. He joined the company in July 2015. Justin's contributions include assisting with the pro–duction of Cannabis medicines, the development of educational materials, and patient care.

Justin's primary interest is the use of Cannabis extracts to treat cancer. He became involved in the field in March 2008, and began rigorously tracking success stories and accumulating the mounting scientific evidence related thereto.

He has presented at several conferences, including the inaugural medical Cannabis events in Australia and Costa Rica, as well as Patients out of Time in 2016.

Justin has also written books on medical Cannabis including *The Comprehensive Report on the Cannabis Extract Movement*, *Enhancing Your Endocannabinoid System*, and *Cannabis for the Treatment of Cancer*. Justin has also written articles for many leading Cannabis-information websites, including Medical Jane.

Elisabeth Mack

Tell me about your journey with Cannabis and your area of expertise.

I found Cannabis in 2015, after crashing my bicycle, needing surgery, and not wanting pain pills. My chiropractor's massage therapist was using CBD in the oils, and that started my journey of discovery.

After I learned how to use it for my acute issues, I started to add CBD and remove prescription medications for my chronic issues. As time progressed, I needed to help others, and established Holistic Caring in 2016, as a nursing case management and educational services firm. Our main focus is chronic or palliative care, with most clients over the age of 70. They most need the help, but so do many 40+ folks who are starting to take medications. Consider Cannabis!

When did your interest in Cannabis start and why?

2015 was a research, study, network, experiment year. I was still working in insurance, but in January 2016, I attended Women Grow national, in Denver. I learned so much about businesses working the supply chain, but no one was sitting down one on one and explaining it to patients. That's what I set out to do because nursing is the missing link.

What are the misconceptions of Cannabis?

People don't want to smoke, and they don't want to be high. They're scared to lose control. They don't want to feel stoned and worry that their life will change along the lines of stereotypes.

Once I assuage their fears, they do fine, and many stay on Cannabis for quite a while. On that note, they also don't want to get addicted. Then, I tell them that Cannabis is a gateway out of addiction – from pills, alcohol, street drugs, workaholism. Cannabis can be a facilitator to health, and people don't know that.

What are the questions you are most frequently asked?

1. Which product do I take?
2. What are ratios of CBD to THC?
3. How much do I take?
4. How often do I take it?
5. What about the other prescription medications that I take every day?
6. What time of day should I take it?
7. Should I eat with it?

What questions should people be asking?

What am I spending on my other prescription medications?
Patients always complain about the cost of Cannabis prescriptions.

What good are the other prescription medications doing for me?
Many times, patients are taking prescription medications that do not help them out of habit or obligation to their doctor, and fear of being without.

How can Cannabis help me improve my quality of life? What is the potential savings in quality of life?
People don't measure the intangibles often enough. Cannabis can get you off the couch, moving, eating better, sleeping better, and more productive.

Should I tell my doctor about it?

Yes. Always make sure the prescriber of other medications knows about Cannabis before you start to reduce other prescriptions.

Should I tell my friends about my Cannabis use?

Yes - they need to hear it from a friend so they can be brave enough to try it for themselves.

What is the recommended starting and titration dosing? Are there any side effects when using Cannabis?

CBD: Begin with 5-10 mgs twice a day, AM or PM, monitor daytime dosing as CBD may be energizing. Increase by 5-10 mgs every week until effects needed are attained. If symptoms worsen, reduce dose by 5-10 mgs and hold a week. Dosing range from 50-200 mgs/day. May see side effects of prescription over 50 mgs. Cancer; up to 5 mgs/kg per day.

1:1 CBD/THC: Begin with 5-10 mgs twice a day, PM or HS. May sedate, add daytime as THC tolerance is built. Increase by 5 mgs every week until effects needed are attained. If symptoms worsen, reduce dose by 5-10 mgs and hold a week. Then, resume and be patient. Max dosing is 50-200 mgs - may see side effects of prescription over 50 mgs. Cancer; up to 5 mgs/kg per day. 3-4/ per day dosing of 1:1 is excellent for opioid weaning.

THC: Begin with 5 mgs as needed in PM or HS. May sedate. Increase by 5 mgs every week until effects needed are attained. If symptoms worsen, reduce dose by 5-10 mgs and hold a week. Then, resume and be patient. Max dosing 50-200 mgs - may see side effects of prescription over 50 mgs. Cancer; up to 5 mgs/kg per day. 1-2 per night dosing of THC.

THC; Dizzy, disoriented, anxiety, intensified awareness, short-term memory impairment, hallucinations, slowed reactions, low blood pressure, low blood sugar, tachycardia, red eyes, broncho-dilation, sedation, muscle relaxation, appetite. CV risk.

CBD; Dizziness, hyperactivity, sedation, loose stools, jitteri-ness, tachycardia

Cytochrome P450 enzymes metabolize Cannabis.

Interactions are possible – especially with 50 mgs or more daily. Be cautious with blood thinners, and watch for synergies with other prescriptions to lower doses. Opiates can be cut in half pretty quickly.

Give me a few examples of a positive experience, benefits, or success stories.

Lorraine was just put on hospice as her daughter contacted me. She has Alzheimer's disease, and was in a care facility on Rem-eron, Seroquel, Ativan, Ambien, Morphine, Zofran, Megace, Dulcolax, and many other prescriptions for blood pressure, heart, and cholesterol.

Lorraine started on a 3:1 tincture, 5 mgs 3-4 times per day. Within 2 weeks, she started to eat and the Megace was cut. After 3 weeks, we changed her to a 1:1 CBD/THC and her Ativan dose was halved and frequency was cut in half. The Seroquel was eliminated after six weeks. She was no longer crying out with anxious fits and her thoughts became more organized.

Seroquel carries a black box warning and the daughter wanted her off of it. After a week, she didn't need the morphine as a rou-tine, and it was only given sporadically. Her cognition cleared more and more with the low doses of 1:1 3-4 times per day, and Lorraine remains on that dose 18 months later.

Patients improve with chronic pain, neuropathic issues, seizures, MS, RA, and autoimmune issues. The key is sustained low doses of very well made medicines. Time heals the body again.

Give me an example for how this is life changing for someone you know.

It's life changing for me! When I crashed my bike, I was on 1800 mgs of Motrin a day, along with 6-8 Flexeril as a muscle relaxant, Fiorinal and Immitrex for migraines, Klonopin for sleep, HCTZ for blood pressure, and Effexor for depression. I had become a widow in 2013, and was struggling with fibromyalgia for 20 years after three shoulder surgeries that fixed nothing. Now I take one Motrin a day. I got my life back.

How has Cannabis helped you/clients/others where other products were unsuccessful?

Traditional medicine is fundamentally flawed. It does well with acute care but can't address chronic care because the body has to heal itself. Functional medicine teachings must accompany the Cannabis medicine. Cannabinoids facilitate movement, mindful eating with anti-inflammatory nutrition, to promote better sleep, and a brighter mood. Traditional antidepressants lack staying power and people have a horrible time coming off of them. Cannabis helps that by stimulating natural production of serotonin and your own endocannabinoid system to work better. Mood regulation is just easier, anxiety drops, and pain improves, along with overall quality of life.

What changes in the industry do you foresee coming in the future?

A continued push towards recreational or adult use Cannabis. This is fine, but a medical model must be saved and promoted because there is so much potential to heal real conditions. Targeted therapies are being developed with terpenes influencing multiple cannabinoid blends of oils. The maturity of product selection in California is mind blowing compared to the primitive markets in the other 33+ states. Standardization must occur so that people can understand general dosing protocols everywhere.

What do you wish people knew or understood about Cannabis?

That this plant is pleiotropic. It can fix many things at once in the body. As you take it for one condition, the other things going wrong also slowly improve. This has a tremendous potential to change the trajectory of medicine in the world, especially America. Because of the endocannabinoid system, adjustments made by supplementing CBD, THC, CBG, THCA, THCV, CBN, and more, we can lower the healthcare spend for prescription medications; pain, anxiety, sleep, appetite, nausea, and mood.

Are there any questions that you feel you would like to address that were not asked?

Where are the healthcare professionals? That question must be asked, and the answer is: hiding. They want to know this is legitimate and need to learn all about Cannabis as medicine. There are now curriculums popping up and I have written training manuals for nurses which I teach at live events. I've also authored *Cannabis for Health: a Guide for Healthcare Professionals.*

We don't need more specialists like myself; we need every provider to be able to have this conversation with patients and for them to be part of the solution instead of perpetuating the problem. As Director of Clinical Operations for True Farma, I am tasked with building a network of qualified professionals across America to help patients.

If you'd like to participate, email me at
emack@truefarma.com.

At the very minimum, read the literature at
www.Cannabisreports.com and www.projectcbd.org as a
fine start.

To your health,
Elisabeth Mack, RN, MBA

Elisabeth Mack, RN, MBA

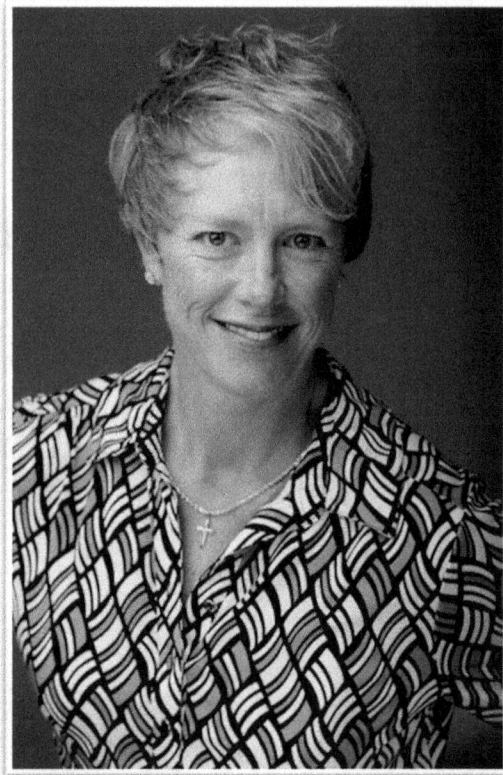

Elisabeth Mack joined True Farma as the Director of Clinical Operations in May 2019, to bridge the gap between traditional and Cannabis medicine. She founded Holistic Caring in 2016, as a concierge medical Cannabis consultation service with clinical nurses helping educate, guide, and support patients with product choices, dosages, and timing. Integrating Cannabis into a treatment plan for complex diseases takes time, knowledge and research that very few practitioners have. Elisabeth professionalizes medical Cannabis at True Farma by equipping providers to have these conversations as part of general patient care.

Elisabeth is a CE education provider for the Board of Registered Nursing developing a Cannabis medicine curriculum to train clinicians, and to teach patients how to approach Cannabis by emphasizing holistic and functional medicine.

Her background includes a decade in hospitals where she specialized in psychiatry, diabetes, and medical units. Elisabeth spent the 20 years prior to Holistic Caring in operations and sales management of several health insurance carriers (RSM of Anthem Blue Cross until 2015), and believes cannabinoid medicine offers our best chance at healing, comfort, and wholeness in a more holistic, economical, and empowering way.

She earned an MBA in Healthcare Administration, a Bachelor of Science in Nursing, and a Bachelor of Arts in psychology.

She is a member of the Society of Cannabis Clinicians, and the American Cannabis Nurses Association.

Jessica Knox, MD MBA MPH; Janice Knox, MD MBA

Tell me about your journey with Cannabis and your area of expertise.

As physicians trained in the allopathic Western medical model, we only learned about Cannabis as a drug of abuse with no medical benefits. As late as 2012, when Drs. Rachel and Jessica graduated from medical school, no information about the medicinal uses of Cannabis, or even about the physiology of the endocannabinoid system (ECS), was included in formal medical education curricula.

In Dr. Jessica's residency training, the only way to formally record a patient's Cannabis use in the electronic medical chart was to code it as "Cannabis use disorder" or "Cannabis abuse." Cannabis use was not only stigmatized in patients, but also in physicians.

Dr. Janice recalls the unfortunate experience of a fellow anesthesiologist who was sent away to rehabilitation due to their use of Cannabis. It was thus thoroughly ingrained in us that Cannabis was nothing but a drug in the most pejorative sense of the word.

It seems almost miraculous then, that not even 10 years after these experiences, all four physicians in our family have become endocannabinologists. In this new discipline, we specialize in the function, dysfunction, and modulation of the ECS. While we remain informed by our conventional specialties - anesthesia for Dr. Janice, emergency medicine for Dr. David, family and integrative medicine for Dr. Rachel, and preventive medicine for Dr. Jessica - we have come to learn and champion the primacy of the

ECS in health and healing. We have also turned our focus to not only managing patients through the lens of the ECS but also to educating our healthcare colleagues and the general public on the existence, function, and modulation of the ECS.

When did your interest in Cannabis start and why?

The Knox doctors' entry into the Cannabis space started with Dr. Janice, who skeptically agreed to cover a colleague's shift at a Cannabis card clinic in 2011. Retired from anesthesia by this time, and a mover and shaker by nature, Dr. Janice had been exploring various avenues to continue promoting health and wellness in her newly found free time. She thought she knew what she'd see at the card clinic - not patients seeking healing, but stoners looking for a doctor's signature so they could get high legally.

That's not what she found. Instead, she saw patients of all ages and walks of life - babies, grandparents, adolescents, adults; students, professionals, retirees; and rich, poor, and everything in between. The only commonality amongst the patients coming through the clinic was that they were all seeking and, more often than not, finding real healing through Cannabis.

With her preconceived notions thus vanquished, Dr. Janice found herself in a new predicament. She—a board-certified anesthesiologist, expert in physiology and pharmacology by training and trade—couldn't answer any of the patients' questions about how Cannabis worked or how they should use or dose it.

Humbled and humiliated, Dr. Janice set about learning all she could about Cannabis. In her efforts, she learned about the fascinating history of Cannabis as a medicine, the sordid history of Cannabis prohibition, the pharmacology and pharmacokinetics of the Cannabis plant, and most importantly, about the incredible system underlying the medicinal effects of Cannabis.

As she pored over books and articles, Dr. Janice shared what she was learning with the rest of us. Just as Dr. Janice was skeptical when she walked through the doors of the Cannabis clinic that first day, we were skeptical at first of what she told us - how could our medical education and training be so wrong? But eventually, our curiosity, our frustration with the conventional medical system and, most movingly, the stories of the patients Dr. Janice was seeing, inspired the rest of us to start reading and learning ourselves. By 2015, all four doctors in the family were practicing in Cannabis clinics at least part-time.

Over the last several years, our collective reading and experiences have shaped for us a new paradigm of medicine - one in which Cannabis is just the tip of an enormous iceberg. While the public conversation remains loudest about the Cannabis plant itself, the true revolutionary subject is the ECS. Certainly, Cannabis is the most versatile herb to affect this system, but it's just one of the many botanical and practical therapeutics that we can use to restore health via the ECS. Widespread knowledge of the ECS will change the way we approach health and disease.

What are the misconceptions of Cannabis?

There are countless misconceptions of Cannabis. The most pernicious of which has been propagated and perpetuated by many top government officials and agencies since the early 20th century - that Cannabis is a drug of abuse with no medical use. This misconception alone has perpetrated immeasurable harm and suffering to people around the world.

Another misconception of Cannabis is that it should only be used as a last resort, when all other medical therapies have failed. Given the plant's broad applicability and remarkably wide safety profile, Cannabis should be considered a first line medication for many conditions and ailments.

A particularly sticky misconception about Cannabis is that it has good phytocannabinoids and bad phytocannabinoids – specifically that CBD is the "good one" and THC is the "bad one." The truth is both CBD and THC have and even share many of the same medicinal benefits. But they also differ in at least one important way: the psychoactive properties of CBD are non-euphoric and non-intoxicating, while the psychoactive properties of THC may cause euphoria or intoxication (the "high"). Rather than being "bad" though, the euphorigenic properties of THC may be therapeutic for some people. Set and setting are incredibly important when administering Cannabis medicine. Who is the person using Cannabis, what are their goals, and in what situation would they be medicating? Informed use of Cannabis can help to optimize the individual's experience. Put differently, there is no bad phytocannabinoid; there is just improper or uninformed use that may lead to a bad Cannabis experience.

What questions are you most frequently asked about Cannabis?

Can I use Cannabis without getting high?

Yes, you can! You can even use THC without getting high if you understand dosing and cannabinoid ratios. In certain ratios to THC, CBD will reduce or prevent the high associated with THC. For naive users, a CBD:THC ratio of 10:1 is typically a good place to start to achieve this synergistic effect while getting the benefits of both phytocannabinoids. This is just one reason why a full spectrum Cannabis product with the full entourage effect in play is preferred.

Can I use Cannabis without smoking?

Absolutely! There are many ways to use Cannabis. Vaporizing, mucosal absorption (e.g., tinctures), ingestibles (e.g., edibles and capsules), topicals, and suppositories are all ways to administer

Cannabis without smoking it. Depending on the patient and their health goals, one method of administration may be better than another, and it may be ideal to even layer multiple methods.

Can Cannabis cure (fill in the blank)?

Cannabis is a multifunctional medical tool that has been found to manage, reverse, or even cure a wide variety of ailments. Unfortunately, we don't have strong clinical trials to verify many of these anecdotal success stories at this time. That said, Cannabis is a remarkably safe medication that has strong anecdotal evidence in its favor - it's almost always worth adding to a therapeutic regimen. In our opinion, it should often be the first line medication in a therapeutic regimen.

Will I become addicted to Cannabis?

Most likely not. Cannabis addiction has been estimated at about 9% of users, and this is likely overstated given the stigma associated with Cannabis and the ease with which the label of addiction has historically been applied to Cannabis users. The vast majority of Cannabis users do not use Cannabis to the detriment of the rest of their lives and can stop using Cannabis whenever they want without physiologic withdrawal symptoms, which means they are not addicted to Cannabis. It's important to contrast these characteristics with Cannabis users who prefer to not stop their Cannabis medication because it successfully manages their chronic illness or because they feel better and more functional while using it.

What is the best way to use Cannabis?

There is no single best way to use Cannabis. Each individual will have their own "best way" to use Cannabis based on their health needs, goals, lifestyle, etc.

What are the five questions people should be asking?

1. What is going wrong in my endocannabinoid system to cause my health concern?

Several of our most troublesome chronic illnesses today have been associated with ECS dysfunction, including obesity, diabetes, rheumatic disease, cancer, migraines, fibromyalgia, irritable bowel syndrome, and PTSD. Ongoing research continues to associate specific ECS dysfunctions with specific disease processes. In order to effectively address, manage, and perhaps reverse or cure a disease, we must understand its root cause. Particularly if you want to use Cannabis in your therapeutic regimen, it's important to understand what is going wrong in your ECS so that you can properly address it.

2. How can I use Cannabis to address my endocannabinoid system dysfunction?

Once the ECS dysfunction is identified, the proper cannabinoid and terpene formulation can be deduced. By considering the patient's other health and lifestyle needs, an appropriate Cannabis regimen can be recommended.

3. What else can I do aside from (or instead of) using Cannabis to address my ECS dysfunction?

The ECS responds to all stimuli to try to keep the body in balance. We can use certain stimuli to help support the ECS in its work. The most important tool (even more important than Cannabis) is nutrition - real, whole foods are our first medicine. Where we can't get all our phytonutrients through food, we can use supplementation to fill the gaps. Detoxifying practices that help to rid our body of toxins can reduce the heavy lifting for the ECS. Activities like moderate exercise, yoga, meditation, acupuncture, chiropractic, and massage also help to stimulate and restore the ECS.

4. How do I use Cannabis safely and responsibly?

Using Cannabis safely and responsibly requires first a basic understanding of how the primary phytocannabinoids work singly and together, how the various administration methods work, and how to apply this information to your health or wellness goals. It's important to know, for instance, that a CBD-dominant medication will protect you from an uncomfortable intoxication experience, that inhaled and mucosal methods work much more quickly than ingested methods, and that low doses are the best place to start.

Another important part of using Cannabis safely is to understand how to read Cannabis products labels so you can choose safe and appropriate medication. You should only use lab-tested products with labels that show the amounts of cannabinoids (and ideally terpenes) present in the product, the serving size and amount of cannabinoids per serving, and the results of contaminant testing - microbes, heavy metals, residual solvents, and pesticides.

Finally, you should make sure to store your Cannabis products securely, especially if you have children or pets in the home - this means out of reach and in childproof packaging.

5. Does it matter what kind of CBD I use?

Yes. Not all CBD and Cannabis products are created equal. Full spectrum products in which the final product accurately represents the full phytochemical profile of the source plant will provide the best efficacy and safest medication experience. This is because the entourage effect - the synergy of each phytochemical constituent working together to create a sum greater than the parts - will be in effect in a full spectrum product. When certain phytochemicals are stripped away to create broad-spectrum, THC-free, or isolate products, the entourage effect is sequentially lost until it's non-existent, leaving a product with less efficacy and a worse safety profile.

Give me a few examples of a positive experience, benefits, or success stories.

An eight-month-old baby was referred to our clinic from a university hospital with a diagnosis of inoperable glioblastoma. The tumor was pressing on the optic nerve causing nystagmus and multiple seizures daily. The young parents were deeply religious and had no experience with Cannabis but were terrified for their baby's life. They hesitantly approached our team for help.

Three months after starting the infant on a Cannabis protocol, the parents saw fewer seizures and scans showed a 25% reduction in tumor size. Six months later, the tumor had reduced in size by 75% and the baby had still fewer seizures and was showing significant gains in his growth and development milestones.

What is the recommended starting dose for clients? Can you overdose? What are the side effects?

The starting dose for Cannabis medicine depends on the individual and the condition being treated. Individuals who are Cannabis-naive will often start with lower doses than those who are Cannabis-experienced. In general, for most people and most conditions, we recommend the age-old medical wisdom of "start low and go slow."

Starting with a micro dose of Cannabis – 2.5 mg to 5 mg per dose – and gradually increasing the dose as needed is smart for a few reasons: (1) it allows the individual to get accustomed to the effects of their Cannabis medicine while minimizing the risk of "overdoing it;" (2) by gradually increasing the dose in small increments only as needed, an individual will find the optimal dose for them – the dose at which they achieve the desired symptom relief without unwanted side effects, aka the minimum effective dose; (3) by starting low and going slow to find their minimum effective dose, the individual is spending their money efficiently, not buying and using more medication than they actually need.

For certain conditions, cancer in particular, specific dose goals do come into play, and these doses are much higher than required for mere symptom relief. Yet even with cancer patients seeking to use Cannabis in their treatment regimen, we recommend starting at relatively low doses and increasing the dose steadily over time so that the body has a chance to acclimate to the medicine while they work up to their therapeutic doses.

There are few to no examples of overdosing with Cannabis in the way we think about drug overdoses, meaning we don't see Cannabis users consuming so much Cannabis that it stops their respiratory drive or any other essential bodily function causing them to die. This happy fact can be attributed to the scarcity of cannabinoid receptors in the brainstem which, among other critical tasks, controls our cardiorespiratory function.

For the most part, overdosing with Cannabis means the user consumed enough to have a bad experience that may include heart palpitations, anxiety, paranoia, panic, and/or feeling that they are going to die. Fortunately, these adverse effects are temporary, wearing off when the high does usually somewhere between 2-10 hours depending on the person and how they medicated. These effects are caused by THC and can be mitigated or avoided altogether with informed use of Cannabis. In the midst of a Cannabis "overdose," typically the only management necessary is to keep the individual as calm and comfortable as possible. Sometimes, administering CBD or the terpenes beta-caryophyllene or limonene can also help reduce THC intoxication.

In the past several years, with spreading legalization of Cannabis and increasing (uninformed) demand for higher THC products, cases of more serious Cannabis overdose requiring temporary respiratory support have arrived to emergency departments. These cases often involve dabbing extremely high THC concentrates or eating too many high THC edibles at once, thereby hitting the body with excessively high THC loads. Again, informed and responsible use (and storage) of Cannabis products can prevent such an overdose experience.

Other side effects of Cannabis may include improved mood, reduced stress, less awkward social interactions, enhanced pleasure, more engaged presence, more interesting conversations, and increased creativity.

Give an example of how Cannabis is/was life changing for someone you know.

Our patients typically come into our clinics with anxiety, insomnia, and pain, all accompanied by extensive drug lists. In many patients, we see a transformation once we find a therapeutic regimen that works for them - less anxiety, improved sleep, and improvement in pain levels. While it's never the explicit goal of therapy, many also have been able to reduce their drug list and get off opioids, which is a moment of pride for a lot of patients.

What changes in the industry do you foresee coming in the future?

As the Cannabis industry edges further into the legal landscape, it will be subject to increasing regulation and standardization. There are both benefits and risks associated with such change. Exercised properly, increasing regulation should result in safer Cannabis products for consumers and patients and economic gains for communities. Increasing standardization should result in Cannabis products that are higher quality, more accessible, and more consistent and reliable.

However, the Cannabis industry is also at risk of becoming the next big business that serves the interests of a wealthy few at the expense of the general public. Federal legalization and rescheduling of Cannabis (which are only a matter of *when* and not *if*) will make way for large companies with deep pockets to finally wade legitimately into the Cannabis space. Without careful regulation, these well-resourced behemoths may push small local businesses out of the industry, doing a major disservice to communities; and if they follow their usual pharmaceutical and consumer goods playbooks, they may flood the market with patented cannabinoid isolates and synthetics of inferior quality and safety, doing a great disservice to consumers and patients.

Avoiding such a grim fate for an industry that is historically rooted in communities, healing, and activism requires knowledgeable and active advocates in the rooms and at the tables where Cannabis policy and regulations are being made. The next few years thus demand a massive education/re-education effort. It is critical that policymakers, regulators, Cannabis cultivators, product manufacturers, Cannabis retail owners and workers, healthcare professionals of every ilk, and members of the general public have at least a basic understanding of how and why Cannabis works. With awareness and advocacy, we reduce our risk of being bamboozled and increase our chances of maintaining an industry that serves the needs of its customers.

What do you wish people knew or understood about Cannabis?

- Cannabis has been used as medicine for millennia. As such, we have abundant evidence that Cannabis is safe. We also have abundant evidence, with growing scientific support, that Cannabis offers significant and broad medicinal benefits.
- Cannabis has been used for food, fuel, and fiber for millennia. Not to mention, it is a fast-growing plant that cleans the soil and air it touches. Cannabis is a multipurpose, eco-friendly plant that could have a massive impact in slowing climate change and reducing pollution.

- Cannabis works as medicine because we have an endocannabinoid system. Cannabis led to the discovery of the ECS, which in turn has reminded us that we have innate healing abilities and instincts that hinge upon our relationships with nature, ourselves, and others.
- Cannabis is but one of the many tools that work to modulate and heal the endocannabinoid system. Other important tools to manage the ECS include nutrition, detoxification, supplementation, physical activity, and healthy relationships.

Are there any questions that you feel you would like to address that were not asked?

CBD and THC are metabolized through the liver's CYP450 system which is also responsible for metabolizing a significant proportion of pharmaceutical drugs. Thus, careful monitoring of pharmaceutical drug levels is highly recommended when using high doses of CBD and THC. Research shows that CBD has a greater effect on the CYP system than THC, which is particularly important to keep in mind as we see CBD become more ubiquitous in the general marketplace.

What are the health benefits related to using Cannabis?

Even a basic understanding of the physiology of the endocannabinoid system helps to explain how Cannabis can be beneficial for so many ailments. The phytocannabinoids produced by Cannabis mimic and modulate the activities of our very own endocannabinoids at cannabinoid receptors, making Cannabis a tool with as broad a range of effects as the functions of the ECS itself.

Cannabis features powerful anti-inflammatory, antioxidant, antitumorigenic, anticonvulsant, antinociceptive, and anxiolytic effects, just to name a few. Here's a quick comparison of some of the benefits of the major phytocannabinoids, CBD and THC:

CBD Benefits	THC Benefits
Analgesia	Analgesia
Anti-inflammatory	Anti-inflammatory
Anti-nausea	Anti-nausea
Anti-tumorigenesis	Anti-tumorigenesis
Muscle relaxation	Muscle relaxation
Anti-oxidant	Anti-oxidant
Anticonvulsant	Anticonvulsant
Anti-anxiety & depression	Antidepressant
Antipsychotic	Neuroprotective

What, if any, are the differences between using CBD vs. THC?

Both CBD and THC are psychoactive, but THC works on CB1 receptors to cause psychotropic effects (the "high"). CBD works allosterically on CB1 receptors, meaning it doesn't bind to them directly but it changes the way they bind to other molecules, including THC. In this way, CBD helps to mitigate some of the typically unwanted side effects of THC that include short-term memory loss, tachycardia, hypotension, anxiety, panic attacks, dry mouth, dysphoria, and motor imbalances.

Do you see research increasing with regards to Cannabis?

Due to Cannabis prohibition in the United States, there are still many unanswered questions about how to best use, dose, and manage Cannabis medicine in humans. Despite these unanswered questions, legalization proceeds and more consumers add some form of Cannabis to their routines every day. Cannabis research is accelerating to answer important clinical questions and to catch up with the legal and social status of the plant. With more research, we hope to see stronger patterns emerge to better inform formulation and dosing guidelines.

That said, it's important to not overlook the absolute abundance of preclinical Cannabis research that has been performed and published dating back to the 1960s. A common refrain amongst the medical establishment is, "there isn't enough research" for clinicians to recommend, or even discuss Cannabis with patients. This is nothing more than a lazy and convenient excuse to avoid the subject. The truth is there are tens of thousands of Cannabis research papers available to inform clinicians working with patients who are already using or asking about Cannabis today. Do we need more research? Of course. Is there already enough research available for clinicians to educate themselves adequately and begin assisting patients? Absolutely.

Are you seeing an increase in medical professionals recommending CBD or other products?

An increasing number of medical professionals are recommending CBD or other Cannabis-based products. Much of this change has come about because patients are driving it. As more and more patients ask their doctors about Cannabis, some doctors are responding responsibly by learning the facts about Cannabis as medicine. Still, other doctors and healthcare professionals are internally motivated to learn about Cannabis as medicine; they are seeking better answers to healing than have been provided by the conventional medical system, and their research often leads them to Cannabis. With a better understanding of Cannabis, and perhaps of the ECS as well, more medical professionals are recommending Cannabis-based products to their patients or, at the least, referring their canna-curious patients to medical professionals who do know.

How can we educate medical professionals about Cannabis and encourage them to consider recommending this to their patients?

The physiology of the endocannabinoid system and the pharmacology of Cannabis must become part of the regular educational curriculum in all medical and allied health schools. It is unconscionable that more than two decades after the identification of the endocannabinoid system, it is still not being taught to students as part of foundational physiology.

Additionally, healthcare professionals need access to science-based and clinically relevant continuing education materials and opportunities. The Knox doctors are doing our part to help fill this need with ADVENT Academy, our training program in clinical endocannabinology and cannabinoid medicine designed for healthcare professionals. We plan to expand our trainings to also fill learning gaps for other direct and indirect stakeholders in the Cannabis industry. As discussed earlier, we all have our part to play in making this industry sustainable and value-driven, which means we all need to be educated.

Finally, we hope to see endocannabinology and cannabinoid medicine become recognized board specialties someday, the same as we recognize anesthesia, emergency medicine, family medicine, and preventive medicine, etc. as specialties today. As a boarded specialty, we will see the development of formal residency and/ or fellowship programs as well as ongoing certification programs in the fields of endocannabinology and cannabinoid medicine.

In the meantime, we encourage medical professionals to embark on the same learning journey we did to get where we are today. Abundant research on the ECS and Cannabis as medicine is out there, available to anyone who cares to find it and read it. In becoming medical professionals, we committed ourselves to lifelong learning in service of our patients. We have already learned a great deal, but we also know there is a great deal more to learn.

JESSICA KNOX

Qualifications: Board certified in Preventive Medicine; co-founder and CEO of the American Cannabinoid Clinics; co-founder of ADVENT Academy; Internationally recognized expert and experienced speaker in Cannabinoid Medicine.

Experience: After completing her residency in preventive medicine, Dr. Jessica Knox began her study of the endocannabinoid system and cannabinoid medicine. She delights in teaching patients, other healthcare professionals, and the public about the power and promise of this incredible system and its associated toolkit. She has spoken on numerous medical Cannabis panels, presented at Cannabis conferences nationwide, and appeared on nationally televised programs and global webcasts to discuss the burgeoning field of endocannabinology.

Dr. Jessica Knox has also developed expertise in the design and delivery of multi-state telemedicine care. During her tenure as medical director at a Silicon Valley telehealth startup, Dr. Jessica oversaw the growth of the telemedicine practice from serving zero patients to over 100,000 patients in just over three years.

Dr. Jessica has a keen interest in health literacy and access. She is CEO and co-founder of The American Cannabinoid Clinics, and co-founder of ADVENT Academy, which offers premier training for the health professional in the ECS, endocannabinology, and cannabinoid medicine. Dr. Jessica serves the Academy as course director, content developer, and lecturer.

Education: Dr. Jessica received her bachelor's degree from Harvard University before going on to earn her medical and business degrees from Tufts University, and her public health degree from San Diego State University.

JoAnn Coleman

Tell me about your journey with Cannabis and your area of expertise?

I am an acute care nurse practitioner currently working as the Clinical Program Coordinator for the Sinai Hospital Center for Geriatric Surgery. I have been a nurse for 45 years and a nurse practitioner for the past 24 years. Most of my professional experience has been with general surgery and surgical oncology patients. I became interested in the surgical care of the older patient 15 years ago when I realized approximately 50% or more of the patients I was caring for were 65 years and older. This number will continue to rise as the population ages and the majority of patients in the hospital become increasingly older in age requiring complex care for multiple morbidities.

When did your interest start in Cannabis and why?

My interest in Cannabis results from questions I pose during the geriatric preoperative assessments I perform. I evaluate patients 75 years and older having any elective surgical procedure. As part of the preoperative evaluation, patients have a review of their medical history, a physical examination, routine laboratory studies and imaging along with medication reconciliation. The focused preoperative geriatric assessments include cognition, function, nutrition, frailty, risk factors for postoperative pulmonary complications, depression screen, hearing screen, fall screen, psychosocial, quality of life assessment, and alcohol and smoking history.

Many older patients also have a number of comorbidities requiring multiple medications. In the smoking history, I include a question about smoking of any product including marijuana. I was definitely intrigued when a number of replies were positive for this question. As part of the medication reconciliation, I ask about the use of Cannabis or any of its products, particularly cannabidiol or CBD. My next consideration was what to tell these patients about using any Cannabis products prior to surgery, especially the night before surgery.

I decided to look at the literature about this question and found there was a deficit of information. I presented the question to the anesthesiologists and nurse anesthetists at my hospital as to what patients should be told about using Cannabis prior to surgery. I found they had little to no knowledge of this issue. I undertook my own research, which incidentally coincided with my state's legalization of medical Cannabis. I researched the state website to learn for what diseases or symptoms medical Cannabis is allowed.

The diseases or symptoms for which medical Cannabis is allowed all coincided with the major chronic medical complaints of the older patient. I discussed the need for better understanding of this new issue with the chief of surgery and he encouraged me to become knowledgeable on the science of medical Cannabis including what is known about both the potential therapeutic benefits, as it may be recommended and administered in the older surgical patient, as well as any harmful or adverse effects.

I reviewed the medical, nursing, and popular literature, attended any conferences for medical professionals that had a talk on the topic, and even attended a conference dedicated to marijuana. I grew more interested and began to share my knowledge with peers and presented at local and national nurse practitioner conferences. The topic of medical marijuana as it relates to the older patient, specifically the older surgical patient, has become my new passion.

What are the misconceptions of Cannabis?

1. People believe that Cannabis only produces euphoria or is used to get high. They have a lack of understanding of the different components of Cannabis and their use for various diseases and symptoms. There is a deficit of information on the endocannabinoid system and its relationship to Cannabis.
2. People may also think that Cannabis is a gateway drug that leads to use of other illicit substances.
3. Another misconception of Cannabis is that it can cure cancer.

What are the five questions you are most frequently asked?

1. What are the interactions between Cannabis and general anesthetic agents and the possible implications for patient care?
2. What research is being done on the effects of Cannabis in the surgical patient, particularly the older surgical patient?
3. What is the role of Cannabis on perioperative complications—cardiopulmonary, coagulation, immunologic, central nervous system?
4. Where can a person find the best evidence-based information about Cannabis use and surgery?
5. Can Cannabis use be combined with opioids postoperatively?

What are the five questions people should be asking?

1. Is it safe to use a Cannabis product prior to surgery? How long before surgery? Should the use of any Cannabis product be stopped prior to surgery and for how long?

2. Have you shared information about your use of Cannabis with your primary care provider or during a preoperative evaluation?
3. What is the evidence-based approach to Cannabis management in the surgical patient?
4. Are there interactions between the prescription and over-the-counter medications one is taking and Cannabis?
5. What is the effect of Cannabis use and surgical considerations of postoperative wound healing, pain management, nutrition?

Give me a few examples of a positive experience, benefits, or success stories.

Older patients having surgery have stated that taking Cannabis has made them less anxious going into surgery. Some have felt they needed less opioid pain medication for treatment of postoperative pain. Other patients stated that they felt their nutritional intake was quicker after surgery.

Give me an example for how Cannabis was life changing for someone you know.

The use of cannabidiol as a sleep aid was invaluable to a family member. There was no longer a need for a medical prescription for a sleep aid.

How has Cannabis helped you/clients/others where other products were unsuccessful?

My family members have benefited from topical Cannabis products for arthritis, which allowed them to be mobile and have a better quality of life with enjoyment of activities and interaction with younger family.

What changes in the industry do you foresee coming in the future?

1. Need for more clinical research into the use of Cannabis and all types of anesthesia.
2. Need for clear guidelines for use of Cannabis before and after surgery.
3. Need for teaching of endocannabinoid system in health professions and the effects of Cannabis.
4. Teach medical Cannabis in pharmacology for all health professionals.
5. Greater dialogue between patient and provider about use of medical Cannabis.
6. Federal government to change the legislation so the medical marijuana industry is the same in every state.
7. Better data collection about use of medical Cannabis during work, driving, personal, and professional time.
8. Follow the same clinical trial procedures that FDA-approved drugs have to pass to be prescribed to patients to dispel myths surrounding Cannabis.
9. Pharmaceutical companies need to come on board and not oppose full-scale legalization for medical marijuana.
10. Medical marijuana as an option instead of another drug.

What do you wish people knew or understood about Cannabis?

It is my wish that individuals understand the risks and benefits of using Cannabis. People must be allowed to consider a Cannabis product as a legitimate option for treatment of a medical problem.

The opportunity for clinical research on Cannabis is boundless. There is much more that is unknown about the use of Cannabis and one must be open to new considerations of its use.

Are there any questions that you feel you would like to address that were not asked?

What information does the surgical community know about the effect of Cannabis on any surgical patient?

Should seniors say yes to Cannabis?

JoAnn Coleman, DNP, ACNP-BC, ANP-BC, AOCN, GCN

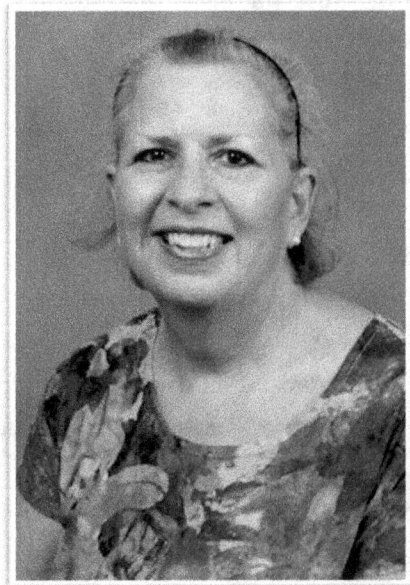

Dr. JoAnn Coleman serves as the Clinical Program Coordinator of the Sinai Center for Geriatric Surgery. She has worked the majority of her professional career caring for surgical patients, from preoperative assessment through postoperative follow-up at The Johns Hopkins Hospital. She has been a clinical nurse, nurse manager, and then a clinical nurse specialist in general surgery. Dr. Coleman's special interests include surgery in the older patient, hepatobiliary and pancreas surgery, transitions in care, and caregiver burden.

As a nurse practitioner since 1996, she has coordinated clinical care of patients, provided education to patients and their families, collaborated on research with surgeons, maintained databases, created critical pathways, lectured locally and nationally, contributed to nursing and medical literature, and mentored graduate and undergraduate nursing students.

Seeing the rise in surgical care of the older patient, Dr. Coleman focused her doctoral studies in this area and was fortunate to find a position that allows her to collaborate with surgeons interested in the care of these patients. She now performs geriatric preoperative assessment for patients 75 years and older having any elective surgery. This assessment includes functional, cognitive and psychosocial assessment, nutritional status, fall and delirium risk, frailty assessment and caregiver burden evaluation.

As a core team member that helped develop the American College of Surgeons Geriatric Surgery Verification program, Dr. Coleman continues on her mission to improve the care of the older surgical patient. Dr. Coleman also helps coordinate The Aging Surgeon Program at Sinai Hospital of Baltimore. This is a comprehensive, objective evaluation of a surgeon's cognitive and physical faculties.

Dr. Coleman is a member of a number of professional organizations including the American Association of Nurse Practitioners, Gerontological Advanced Practice Nurses Association, American Association of Critical-Care Nurses, American Geriatrics Society, and the American College of Surgeons.

Michael Williams

Tell me about your journey with Cannabis and your area of expertise?

My journey into Cannabis started with investigation into the science of cannabinoids, specifically the therapeutic benefits of cannabidiol (CBD) and associated cannabinoids on both the human body and mind.

When did your interest in Cannabis start and why?

In 2017, I was leading a team of neuroscientists and data science professionals creating artificial intelligence and machine learning algorithms to analyze hyper and hypo blood flow in the brain with a focus on predicting early detection of neurological diseases including Alzheimer's, Dementia, and Parkinson's. I first heard about and saw evidence of the application of cannabinoids on both neurological diseases and soft tumors during a private webinar with internal scientists and experts in pharmacology at one of the largest healthcare research institutions. The results were astounding and enough to spark my full-time interest into how Cannabis could be used to address these conditions at a scientific and healthcare level.

What are the misconceptions of Cannabis?

It seems that when people hear the term Cannabis, they think of marijuana and getting high when, in fact, tetrahydrocannabinol (THC), which is the cannabinoid that gives users a euphoric feeling or, "high" is just one of over 100 cannabinoids identified in the Cannabis sativa plant. As more and more research is conducted, scientists are finding tremendous therapeutic benefits using different combinations of cannabinoids.

What are the five questions you are most frequently asked?

We specialize in making CBD Nano Emulsions, so I get questions about CBD in general and then more scientific questions regarding Nano Emulsions, bioavailability, and the best ways to consume Cannabis.

1. What are Nano Emulsions?

Often marketed as "Nano Enhanced CBD" or "Water Soluble CBD," nano CBD is created when CBD oil is processed through highly specialized nano-emulsification systems. This process decreases the size of particles small enough that they can be absorbed directly into the body passing through the digestive system through the epithelial cells of the small intestine. Our proprietary manufacturing process reduces the size of cannabinoids to less than 20 nanometers dramatically increasing bioavailability and absorption into the body and making it the most effective way to use and benefit from CBD. We also use a laser diffracting particle size analyzer for quality control and third-party testing to ensure the best quality product. You can see the difference in quality with the naked eye and in a simple water test.

2. How are CBD Nano Emulsions made?
3. Do they really increase absorption of bioactive lipids (CBD) by 600% into the human body when ingested?
4. Is it a proven technology?
5. What are the five questions people should be asking?

Is the product I am putting into my body safe, is it organic and all natural? What should I look for when choosing the right products?

Like with any other product, you should check the labels for natural ingredients. Look for broad spectrum CBD nano emulsions. Most companies use isolate, and some even sell micro-emulsions or liposomes and pass them off as nano emulsions. When looking for high quality vs. low quality nano CBD, a water test is the easiest way to test liquid nano CBD for clarity and quality. Put a serving of CBD into a bottle or glass of water and check for clarity and taste.

High-quality nano will look like lemonade in its natural state and "translucent" before adding into water or other beverages where it should be clear. Poorly-formulated nano will be cloudy or mildly cloudy; this is a reflection of poor formulation, processing, and large particle sizes.

Other important items to look for are:

- Is the CBD is Water Soluble?
- Is the CBD Colloidal?
- Is the CBD full spectrum CBD (not isolate)?
- No non-synthetics used
- No petroleum synthetics used
- No ethanol/solvents used in processing
- No cellulose encapsulation
- No crystalline used
- Uses only certified organic ingredients for solubility
- How fast does it absorb?

What are the recommended ways of consuming cannabinoids and what consumption methods should be avoided?

Generally, vaping = bad and ingesting = good.

Ingesting is the easiest and least harmful way to consume CBD. Our bodies can process the CBD effectively without doing other harm to the body unlike vaping the product.

Does the product I am consuming come with third-party testing for things like pesticides and heavy metals?

Ask for copy of any testing (certificate or analysis) done on the CBD, and the nano emulsion after it has been processed. A third-party batch test for products for heavy metals, microbes, pesticides, herbicides, cannabinoids and terpenes, and VOC's. Most companies will post their COA testing on their website. Our products are tested at least 2-3 times before they are marketed. I would not trust the product if the company cannot provide proof of testing.

How much of what I am ingesting is being absorbed and utilized by my body? Why is bioavailability important?

Bioavailability refers to how much of a substance is actually absorbed and utilized by the body. A process known as "first pass metabolism" is where the digestive system and liver remove anything that it thinks is toxic (Google: first pass metabolism) before entering the bloodstream. With standard CBD oil, for example, first pass metabolism removes approximately 87-94% of traditional CBD before it is absorbed into the bloodstream. This means that, 90% of the product never reaches a user's system, and is wasted.

For example, if a user ingests 10 mg of traditional CBD oil, only 1 mg or so is actually absorbed and utilized by the body. Because of the smaller particle sizes, nano-emulsified CBD is absorbed into the body approximately 600% more efficiently than traditional CBD oil when ingested. This increase in absorption means that users get 6x the benefits from the same serving size. The uptake and effect is felt within 5 minutes vs. 30 or more minutes with traditional oil-based products.

When ingesting traditional CBD oil, only about 6%-10% actually makes it through the digestive system and into the bloodstream, meaning that about 90% is wasted and not utilized by our bodies. The water soluble cannabinoid nano emulsions we produce get absorbed into the body about 600%+ more effectively than the same amount of CBD Oil. (10 mg CBD oil is equivalent to 60 mg of CBD nano emulsion.)

What is the recommended starting and titration dosing? Are there side effects or concerns when using Cannabis?

We recommend that consumers start with a low serving size and gradually increase based on how their body reacts and what indication they are taking it for. In general, someone taking Cannabis for pain could start treatment at a higher level than someone using it for long-term health benefits. GW Pharmaceutical, whose FDA-approved product is used for treating seizures in children, recommends starting with 2.5 mg twice a day and increasing to 10 mg twice per day. While the industry recommends 10 mg for adults, it's not uncommon for people to take 100 mg or more per day. Also, higher milligrams per bottle is not necessarily better. Nano CBD emulsions are more effective and use less per serving than traditional CBD therefore saving you money by requiring less mg per serving.

Give me a few examples of a positive experience, benefits, or success stories.

Working in the Cannabis industry gives me direct access to patients whose lives have been changed for the better by using Cannabis. One of the most dramatic examples I have seen firsthand is a friend's dog who has cancer and was given three months to live. His owners administer 10 mg of cannabinoids twice a day and he is doing great (18 months later). The benefits of nano emulsion CBD for animals is that it is easier for their bodies to consume. Many animals are sensitive to the oil which can cause other side effects (vomiting, nausea, and drowsiness). Research is still being done on the effects of CBD on animals. I suggest asking your veterinarian for guidelines on how to effectively dose your animal.

Another example is, my friend Scott lives with chronic pain and he was severely depressed. When he switched to nano emulsion CBD, the effects of taking Cannabis to help manage his illness was immediate. He was able to ingest less product and get a faster and more effective result than with any other product. He was able to function during the day without the drowsy effects of other drugs. He is now off opioids and is just one happy fucking camper.

Give an example for how Cannabis was life changing for someone you know.

I have personally seen positive effects in an elderly gentleman who has Parkinson's disease. Within one week of starting a daily regimen of 25 mg of CBD, his symptoms dramatically reduced including less shaking, better sleep, increased cognitive function, and less depression. He was able to decrease his other medications and is living a better life because of cannabinoids.

How has Cannabis helped you/clients/others where other products were unsuccessful?

I regularly receive feedback from consumers of our products who have successfully discontinued use of opioids and other pharmaceutical pain medications. This offers nonscientific evidence that cannabinoids in fact have a strong analgesic effect on the human body. Currently, research on the different cannabinoid is being studied to determine which specific strains are more effective for sleep, pain, and overall health.

Sleep is another big factor. More and more research is being done that shows the importance of getting good sleep. Several people close to me use cannabinoids to help them successfully get a good night's rest, which in turn helps the body deal with other health issues in a much more effective way.

What changes in the industry do you foresee coming in the future?

As more clinical trials are completed, we will see pharmacology advance the use of cannabinoids to treat very specific healthcare issues. Currently, all we know is that the combination (the "entourage effect") of cannabinoids work in a synergistic manner across a large variety of indications. Researchers are on the tip of the proverbial iceberg when it comes to figuring out how and why cannabinoids are effective at treating so many different conditions.

As the stigma of "marijuana" fades, use of cannabinoids will become mainstream and in 10 or 20 years, the next generation will view Cannabis in a very different way than generations before them.

What do you wish people knew or understood about Cannabis?

There are several different drug delivery systems i.e., vaping, ingesting, smoking, and injecting. Most of these are to avoid what is known as "first pass metabolism" which is where the body removes anything it thinks is toxic before letting it into your bloodstream. Several of these methods are extremely harmful to our bodies; for example, vaping oil or flavored e-cigarette-based products into our lungs does bad things. Our lungs are amazing, but they were not created to filter oil-based particles.

In the coming years, we will hear more and more bad stories surrounding vaping, just like we did with cigarettes. Currently, several states have banned the use of flavored e-cigarettes and vaping. Our bodies are not designed to process the artificial chemicals that are in these products. My advice is to do your research and find effective ways to use Cannabis which do not harm the body. Ingesting, for example, seems to be the least harmful way to take advantage of all the good things in Cannabis.

Michael Williams
CEO 5280 Nano Technologies

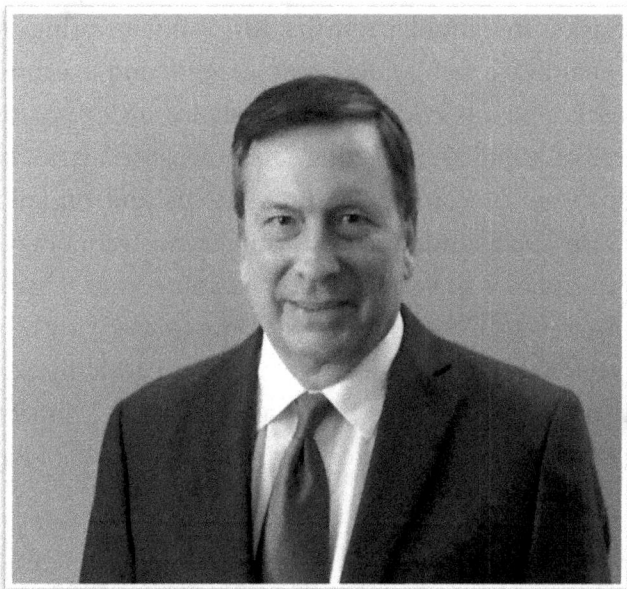

Before devoting his work fulltime and prior to founding 5280 Nano Technologies, Mr. Williams was focused on Artificial Intelligence (AI) and multi-variate statistical machine learning in computational based health algorithms with an emphasis on detecting neurological diseases including Alzheimer's, dementias, and traumatic brain injury. Leading a team of neuroscientists, data scientists, and software engineers committed to understanding how neurological diseases could be addressed "outside of the box", prompted his interest in alternative medicine and specifically how cannabinoids could be used to treat healthcare issues affecting humans with acute and chronic pain. After investigating the efficacy of cannabinoids used to treat a wide variety of health issues, he decided to focus his energy on the most effective and most bioavailable way of introducing cannabinoids into the human body for clinical heterogeneity, including by indication, cannabinoid, and outcome. The result has been the creation of CBD nano emulsions which offer the scientifically highest bioavailability and therapeutic benefits of any drug delivery system.

Focused on shareholder returns, Mr. Williams brings over 30 years of healthcare technology management and executive acumen to each business challenge with his intrinsic flair for innovation, creative problem solving, and measured risk-taking to drive consistent bottom-line improvements and organic value creation. He has founded several successful technology based start-up companies in various domains and acts as a trusted advisor to numerous Cannabis related companies giving advice on evidence based medicine, growth tactics, and go-to market strategies. As a C-Level executive, he has been a key contributor in creating exits generating in excess of $650M in shareholder value.

Dr. Abhishek Rai

Disclaimer: The below excerpt is not based on clinical expertise and simply highlights my understanding of the Cannabis plant. Anything that I have mentioned in this chapter should not be taken as a clinical recommendation by a physician. Most of my opinions are based on my understanding of Western literature and of Eastern Ayurvedic Medicine and statistical data available.

Tell me about your journey with Cannabis and your area of expertise? When did your interest in Cannabis start and why?

My area of expertise is psychiatry. My home country is India, which has a potpourri of cultural beliefs. One among those beliefs include Cannabis as one of the five most sacred plants on earth. My first encounters with Cannabis was in the form of green tinged sweets that were available and bought on Maha Shivratri and Holi (two pretty well-known Indian festivals) every year. The sweets were kept way out of our reach as children, which made me very curious. However, I never really got to lay my hands on the "Bhang" form of Cannabis laden treats, but my curiosity persisted.

Vedic literature discusses three therapeutic parts of the Cannabis plant. "Bhang" is a name for the leaves of male and female plants. "Ganja" refers to the flowering tops of the female plant, and "Charas" is the name for the plant resin which naturally exudes from the leaves, stems, and fruits of plants that grew in the Himalayan mountains.

Folklore tells us that the Hindu gods churned the cosmic ocean to obtain Amrit, the elixir of immortality. Cannabis plants grew wherever the drops of this elixir fell on Earth, which is quite telling about its status as a miracle plant. In a different version of the mythological tales, Shiva was summoned to drink the poison from the churned ocean, his throat turned blue (Neelkanth), and the agony of the burning poison was too much to handle. His consort, goddess Parvati, churned some "Bhang" and he was then relieved of the pain. Much of the medicinal lore around "Bhang" comes from such stories where Lord Shiva uses the plant to cure an ailment.

My family is very spiritual, and I can safely say, rationally religious. I always found a harmonious amalgamation of science, religion, and spirituality in my family. My dad, an engineer, advocated logic and reason at all times, and my mom added just the right blend of religious and spiritual beliefs to our family of four. We used to visit ashrams of our "Guru," AKA, teacher. At the ashrams, I saw the use of Cannabis, among other herbs, for healing and spiritual purposes. When I asked questions about use of Cannabis and other herbs used in the ashram, I was told the miracle plant was a divine gift from gods and the concoctions being the products of years of research by holy, wise, guardian figures known as sages.

The mythology around the benefits of drinking "Bhang" for health and success has sparked much interest over thousands of years. In the Vedic texts, "Bhang" is said to help in the treatment of a variety of medical conditions, from epilepsy to depression and in recent years, THC oil has been used effectively by scientists for the same. Particularly in northern India, "Bhang" is believed to be an omen of success; a dream of bhang is seen as a telling sign of future prosperity.

The myths origin cannot be traced, but they remain a part of the ever-evolving aura that surrounds the consumption of "Bhang" in India. Ultimately, *Bhang* is a physical manifestation of Shiva's deepest philosophy which states, "that which can destroy can also create."

Time passed, and I became a medical student. Medical school has a unique way of molding our perspective and creating internal conflicts. My left brain considered Cannabis the villain in the world of evidence-based annals of western medicine and my right brain still maintained my curiosity and held the attention for years. My right brain and my left brain were in conflict about the miracle plant throughout most of my life. The internal discord and my curiosity for the medicinal qualities of this herb encouraged me to obtain a certification in Ayurveda.

Ayurveda has literature suggesting the application of the medicinal properties of Cannabis in various well-recognized medical conditions. Certain extracts and forms of Cannabis can be helpful in treating various medical problems and also helpful in the treatment for mental health symptoms of anxiety and insomnia.

History of Cannabis.

Cannabis is believed to be one of the oldest plants to exist in human history. It has been mentioned in almost all of the ancient history. Cannabis is very familiar throughout central Asia and the Indian subcontinent.

Medical journals across the world focus on the different uses of Cannabis. One for reference is the Chinese medical journal written by Chinese Emperor Shen Nung, known as the Father of Chinese Medicine, around 2700 B.C. talked about benefits of Cannabis. Other ancient documentation includes ancient papyrus from Egypt to include Cannabis as a useful treatment for inflammation.

Arab and other cultures have used marijuana recreationally while other substances like alcohol consumption was banned by the Koran.

In terms of mental health, most of the scriptures describe Cannabis being used for anxiety and sleep problems. There are several mentions of prolonged and heavy use of Cannabis leading to a hallucination-like state where the "devil's eye" can be seen. There is extensive mention of Cannabis being used for attaining spiritual awakening while on the path of self-discovery. It was believed to bring you closer to God.

STATS ON CANNABIS.

The Substance Abuse and Mental Health Services Administration (SAMHSA) (2018) conducted a national survey on drug use and health. Results suggested an estimated 43.5 million Americans aged 12 or older in 2018, used marijuana in the past year. This number of past-year marijuana users corresponds to 15.9 percent of the population. The percentage of the population in 2018, who used marijuana was higher than the percentages from 2002 to 2017. This increase in marijuana use among people aged 12 or older reflects increases in marijuana use among both young adults aged 18 to 25 and adults aged 26 or older.

As per the same report from SAMHSA, marijuana use disorder occurs when someone experiences clinically significant impairment caused by the recurrent use of marijuana, including health problems, persistent or increasing use, and failure to meet major responsibilities at work, school, or home. Survey respondents who used marijuana on six or more days in the past 12 months were categorized as having a marijuana use disorder if they met the DSM-IV criteria for either dependence or abuse for marijuana.

Approximately 4.4 million people aged 12 or older in 2018, had a marijuana use disorder in the past year, which corresponds to 1.6 percent of the population (SAMHSA, 2018). The percentage of the population aged 12 or older in 2018, with a marijuana use disorder was similar to the percentages in most years between 2002, and 2017.

The collected and presented data reflect that a large portion of the United States population is using Cannabis while at the same time, a significant population in America is misusing Cannabis.

Before getting into the details of use and misuse of Cannabis in the mental health field, let's gain some knowledge into the two big constituents of Cannabis. The two main identified components in Cannabis are THC and CBD. The cannabinoid tetrahydrocannabinol (THC) is well known for its psychoactive properties, and cannabidiol (CBD), the second-most abundant component, is the non-psychoactive component of the plant. THC and CBD concentration varies in different plants. CBD is believed to balance a lot of psychoactive adverse effect of THC. THC is mind activating at low and moderate doses. At a high dose, THC is hallucinogenic in nature.

Different strains of the plant have different amounts of THC and CBD. Hemp plants have high levels of CBD that can be extracted to make oil, but marijuana plants grown for recreational use have higher concentrations of THC compared with CBD. Cannabis plants grown for industrial purposes must contain lesser concentrated levels of THC to be considered legal and be marketed as CBD.

Cannabis and its use in mental health is still something that's mostly handled by certain group of psychiatrists who believe in Integrative Psychiatry or have some training in Ayurveda. Western Medicine has not identified clear guidelines on benefits of Cannabis in mental health symptoms and diagnosis. The Cannabis plant and different forms is still considered a recreational substance.

The National Academies of Sciences, Engineering, and Medicine (2017), highlights and discusses the following six mental health diagnosis. The article divides each mental health diagnosis into two categories first being "does Cannabis use lead to development of a mental health diagnosis" and second "how does regular use affect the course and symptoms of already existing mental health diagnosis?"

1.a Cannabis Use and the Development of Anxiety Disorders

The report deliberated that there is limited evidence between Cannabis use and the development of any type of anxiety disorder, except social anxiety disorder. They reported moderate evidence of correlation between regular Cannabis use and increased incidence of social anxiety disorder.

1.b Cannabis Use and the Course or Symptoms of Anxiety Disorders

The report suggested limited evidence of correlation between near-daily Cannabis use and increased symptoms of anxiety.

2.a Cannabis Use and the Development of Schizophrenia or Other Psychoses

The 2017, National Academy report suggested there is substantial evidence of association between Cannabis use and the development of schizophrenia or other psychoses, with the highest risk among frequent users.

2.b Cannabis Use and the Course or Symptoms of Schizophrenia or Other Psychoses

When it comes to psychotic disorders, cognitive dysfunction is a core feature of schizophrenia. Deficits are moderate to severe across several domains, including attention, working memory, verbal learning and memory, and executive functions.

The report suggested moderate evidence that, among individuals with psychotic disorders, the history of Cannabis use was associated with better cognitive performance (better learning and memory task).

3.a Cannabis Use and the Development of Bipolar Disorder or Mania

As per the report, there is limited evidence of an association between Cannabis use and the likelihood of developing bipolar disorder, particularly among regular or daily users.

3. b Is there an association between Cannabis use and the course or symptoms of bipolar disorder?

There is moderate evidence of an association between regular Cannabis use and increased symptoms of mania and hypomania in individuals diagnosed with bipolar disorders.

4.a Cannabis Use and the Development of Depressive Disorders or Symptoms

There is moderate evidence of an association between Cannabis use and a small increased risk for the development of depressive disorders.

4.b Cannabis Use and the Course or Symptoms of Depressive Disorder

There is no evidence to support an association between Cannabis use and changes in the course or symptoms of depressive disorders.

5.a Cannabis Use and Suicidal Ideation, Suicide Attempts, and Suicide

There is moderate evidence of an association between Cannabis use and increased incidence of suicidal ideation and suicide attempts, with a higher incidence among heavier users. The report also added that there is moderate evidence of an association between Cannabis use and increased incidence of suicide completion.

6.a Cannabis Use and the Development of PTSD

There is no evidence to support or refuse an association between Cannabis use and the development of posttraumatic stress disorder.

6.b Is There an Association Between Cannabis Use and the Course or Symptoms of PTSD

There is limited evidence of an association between Cannabis use and an increased severity of posttraumatic stress disorder symptoms among individuals with posttraumatic stress disorder.

Contrary to the above conclusions that were presented by the National Academy, there are few symptoms in which a small case series and clinical trials have shown benefits of Cannabis among patients with PTSD, insomnia and anxiety.

Elms, Shannon, Hughes, and Lewis (2019), concluded that administration of CBD in oral form, and routine psychiatric care displayed a reduction in PTSD related symptoms. The study also suggested that CBD offered other symptom reduction in patients with PTSD including self-reports of nightmare.

Similarly, Shannon, Lewis, Lee and Hughes (2019), identified additional impacts of CBD on mental health symptoms including anxiety and insomnia. The authors reported that 72 adult participants that were identified with anxiety and poor sleep, self-reported sleep scores and anxiety scores decreased within the first month of the study involving administration of CBD.

What are the misconceptions about Cannabis?

Cannabis is a plant that has multiple constituents which are extracted from different parts of the plant. The biggest misconception arises when people make a blanket statement based on their personal experience including:

"Cannabis is very good/bad for anxiety"
"Cannabis is very good/bad for PTSD"
"Cannabis is very good/bad for depression"

These statements should not be absolute in light of the currently documented research on this subject. Misconceptions arise when you don't know your body, your mental state, and your spiritual awareness. My experience and knowledge of Ayurveda has taught me that every individual is different and needs a healing process very much catered to their physical body constituent (Dosha), Mind (Manas) and Spirit (Atman). When you pay attention to your mind, body, and soul to make a conscious decision customized to your needs, there is no place for judgment or misconception concerning your healing.

What questions are you most frequently asked?

I am frequently asked by patients, friends, and acquaintances about the pros and cons of Cannabis. Through experience, I can tell you that people are very opinionated when it comes to the use of Cannabis. Most questions I am asked are to determine if I agree or disagree with preconceived notions. Below are a few statements that are usually stated to me:

- "I take Cannabis because it helps me with my anxiety."
- "I take Cannabis because it helps me to sleep."
- "I use Cannabis because it's better than using alcohol and other drugs."
- "Cannabis is not a drug because you do not have withdrawals from it" or "You cannot overdose on it. "

What questions should people be asking?

Questions about "What people should be asking about Cannabis?" should be no different than the questions we ask ourselves when putting anything else in our body. I would recommend people understanding their body and becoming more aligned with their five senses. Five questions you should be asking are:

- "Am I listening to my body and being mindful of my choice to use Cannabis?"
- "Am I aware of my intention of choosing to use Cannabis?"
- "Am I aware of what I am consuming is part of a nature and eventually will become part of me?"
- "Am I aware of the source of the food I am consuming?"
- "Am I aware of how much should I consume?"

What changes in the industry do you foresee coming in the future?

I think changes are already happening at a very fast pace in the Cannabis industry. I would predict more research conducted in the field of mental health and Cannabis use. The research will be more catered to THC and CBD use. Cannabis is considered a mainstream treatment modality in the Eastern Medicine, Ayurveda. I would hope to see a more blended approach including Western Medicine and Integrative Psychiatry.

I also see it becoming a significant part of Western Medicine and, hopefully, mainstream in the field of Integrative Psychiatry.

What do you wish people knew or understood about Cannabis?

I wish people would have clear intention and awareness when they use Cannabis. I feel people fall prey to peer pressure and most of the time blindly believe popular stories and notions about the herb without genuine verification. People should have better insight of their physical and spiritual self. As I mentioned from my early years, people who I feel have gained the most from Cannabis are the yogic practitioners in the ashram I visited with my family.

People should be aware of their own body and self-health before they turn to Cannabis and then reach out to a reliable authorized provider. I think it's very important to use Cannabis under the supervision of a provider as compared to recreational consumption. You should do "self-reflection" and evaluate yourself honestly to determine if consumption of Cannabis is a short-term fix for your problems (Band-Aid solution), or is it going to help you in long term?

I strongly recommend reaching out to an Ayurveda practitioner because they have the most knowledge in healing with herbs. Being a Western Medicine practitioner and having closely studied Eastern Medicine, I recommend talking to an Integrative Psychiatrist for suggestions about the use of Cannabis for mental health therapies. I still think Cannabis will take time to become mainstream in Western Psychiatry. Western Medicine is supported by evidence-based research and data collection. In order for Cannabis to be mainstream in the future, it will require additional research and Food and Drug Administration (FDA) approval, which will take time.

Abhishek Rai, MD

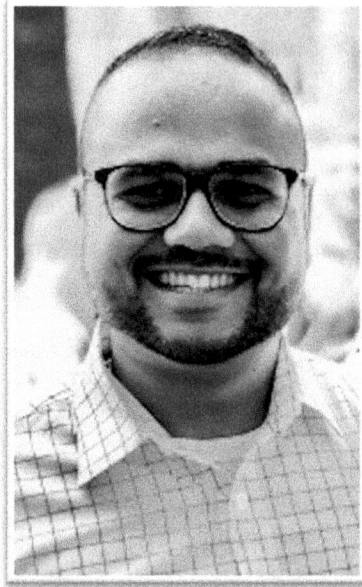

Dr. Abhishek Rai, MD is a full-time American Board of Psychiatry and Neurology certified psychiatrist in California. After graduating from medical school at Delhi University (University College of Medical Sciences) in India, he moved to the USA. In a brief stint at the Mayo Clinic in Rochester, MN (2010-2011), he gained first-hand experience in the department of psychiatry.

After that, he joined the child psychiatry unit of New York State Psychiatry Institute (Columbia University). He moved to Michigan thereafter to complete his post-graduation degree in psychiatry. After completing his residency, he worked at University of Pittsburgh Medical Center for three years and served as the Medical Director in his last year at UPMC. Dr. Rai continues to work with University of Pittsburgh as a volunteer Clinical Assistant Professor of Psychiatry.

Dr. Rai is a member of the American Psychiatric Association. He has many psychiatric publications to his credit and has presented several posters and cases on different psychiatric disorders at the national and international level. He has made prolific contributions to Integrative Psychiatry through his meticulous analysis of "Ashwagandha" and its employment in enhancing and supplementing the mental health treatments currently available. He has presented webinars on yoga and its impact on prevention and treatment of mood disorders. During his term at University of Pittsburgh, Dr. Rai also completed a research study on effects of MBSR on stress level of behavioral health employees.

Dr. Rai also completed a certification course in Eastern Medicine (Ayurveda) from the California college of Ayurveda as he firmly believes in integration of Ayurvedic and Allopathic Medicine for the better prevention and healing of chronic disease.

"The Health Effects of Cannabis and Cannabinoids: The Current State of Evidence and Recommendations for Research." Washington, DC: The National Academies Press. https://doi.org/10.17226/24625.

Dr. Sarah Silcox

Tell me about your journey with Cannabis, your area of expertise, and how you became interested in Cannabis.

I am a small animal veterinarian (meaning I deal predominately with dogs and cats), and am a founding director and the current president of the Canadian Association of Veterinary Cannabinoid Medicine.

When I started practicing 20+ years ago, I had a keen interest in what at that time was known as complementary and alternative medicine. After several years in general practice, I opened a house-call practice that provided an integrative approach to health care. This meant that in addition to the treatments commonly used in practice, I also provided natural diet consultations, homeopathy, chiropractic, acupuncture, laser therapy, as well as nutritional supplements and herbal medicine. So, I suppose that attracted the type of clients that would also be most interested in using Cannabis for their animals.

Around the time that I started seeing patients who were receiving Cannabis from the owners, I had also started spending a lot of time in Jamaica visiting my best friend who was had lived there for five years. During my visits, I became intrigued about the use of Cannabis from a medical point of view. I was fascinated by the Jamaican herbalists who discussed its wide array of actions and the elders who would make tea at night to "help settle the nerves."

As a veterinarian with a keen interest in natural medicines, I began to investigate if Cannabis could help our patients as well and was surprised to find a vast amount of research using animals that suggested it could.

So, while I was far from what I'd call an "advocate," I was canna-curious from a medical point of view, and closely followed my patients who were receiving Cannabis with a great deal of interest. Where possible, I provided guidance to my clients to ensure that my patients were as safe as possible and unlikely to experience any adverse side effects.

One day, I received a call from someone organizing a Cannabis conference and asked if I would participate in a panel discussion on "Pot for Pets." While I had spent my entire adult life avoiding public speaking events, the topic was so interesting, I felt the pull to participate. Besides, she said it would be very informal, just a group sitting on stage in chairs and having a discussion. It sounded good. But, two weeks before the event, there were no other speakers. Petrified that I would be on stage alone, I called everyone I could think of to see if they would join me.

On one such call, I was asked, "Is there a group that is currently advocating for veterinarians on this topic?" and I said, "No, but there should be." And, somehow that went from a casual question to me stating on stage at the conference that we were starting a non-profit to advocate for the use of medical Cannabis for pets. And, once it was said out loud, we made it happen.

The Canadian Association of Veterinary Cannabinoid Medicine is now a leading voice on the use of Cannabis for animals, conducts educational events across the country, and is actively engaged in advocacy work to ensure that veterinarians can provide Cannabis as a medical option for our patients.

What are the misconceptions of Cannabis?

After almost a century of prohibition of Cannabis, it should be no surprise that there are a LOT of misconceptions about Cannabis. I feel that veterinary medicine is the one area where there is still a lot of misinformation surrounding THC.

With the growing interest in CBD and its benefits, THC has become demonized. Yes, we see a lot of dogs presenting in distress due to THC intoxication, but this is almost always due to over-consumption.

With appropriate education and veterinary oversight, I believe THC as part of the total cannabinoid treatment plan can offer many potential benefits.

It is reasonable to expect that THC holds the potential to aid many animals, just as it has proven beneficial for many human patients. However, like most medications, the "poison is in the dose," so we must be more diligent about educating our clients and more cautious with its use to avoid putting our patients at risk.

What are the five questions you are most frequently asked?

1. Can Cannabis help my pet?
2. What dose should we use?
3. Are CBD pet products legal?
4. (from veterinarians) What can we discuss with our clients who ask about Cannabis?
5. Is there science to support the use of Cannabis in veterinary practice?

What five questions should people be asking?

1. Considering both the risks and potential benefits, is Cannabis a reasonable treatment to add to my pet's current treatment plan?
2. Do I need to adjust any other medications that my pet may be taking, or be aware of potential drug interactions?
3. What type of Cannabis product would be best suited in this situation? This could include format (oil, capsule,

treats), cannabinoid profile (THC:CBD, minor cannabinoids), as well as terpene profile (terpenes removed or
included?, predominant terpenes included?)

4. Where should I be purchasing my products and what
should I be looking for in a Cannabis product?

5. How should I begin treatment, what signs should I be
monitoring, and when should I arrange my next follow-
up with my veterinarian?

*Give me a few examples of a positive experience, benefits, or
success stories.*

I have several great stories, but one of my favorites is the story
of Trek. Trek is an amazing dog who lives with an amazing family. He served as a guide dog for his visually-impaired human
for many years before being retired shortly before his 11th birth-
day.

He had worked through allergies, hypothyroidism, a thyroid
tumor (that was successfully surgically removed while still small),
and early arthritis.

I was called out to see Trek one day because he had all but
stopped eating. His weight had dropped significantly, and when
he greeted me at the door, my gut told me this was not good. He
had gone from an active, fit Labrador, to what can only be described as emaciated. For almost a month, his appetite had been
declining, and now he was barely eating anything at all, and certainly not his usual meals. A physical exam and a battery of
blood tests were performed showing several *minor* changes; each
one on their own not overly concerning, but I was still concerned.

We arranged for Trek to see a specialist who performed an
abdominal ultrasound and found abnormalities on both his
spleen and liver. No definitive diagnosis was made, and his family decided not to pursue biopsies at that time, but the specialist

sent him home with several medications to help control nausea and improve his appetite.

However; two weeks later, there was little improvement in Trek at all. We added some additional medications to his regimen, but over the next week, he continued to only pick at treats. I remember that visit clearly; it was almost two months since his appetite started to decline, and three weeks from his visit with the specialist. We sat on the couch, and we both cried knowing that without improvement, Trek would continue to waste away. We had the difficult discussion about how far they were willing to go, and at what point they would be prepared to say goodbye.

At some point during that discussion, Cannabis came up. While we did not have a definitive diagnosis, and we knew little about how it may affect him, we decided that, given the options, it was worth a try. By this point, Trek's appetite had been off for almost two months, and we had been trying various combinations of medications for over three weeks with little improvement. And so, the next day, Trek's family started giving him small amounts of medical Cannabis oil – one high in CBD and very low in THC. That was on a Thursday. He had a little more on Friday, and little more on Saturday, and Sunday morning he went to his food bowl and ate. I was out to see him for a scheduled follow-up that Monday, and when I arrived, the mood in that house had completely changed. I was greeted by a smiling client and tail-wagging Trek, with the news that he had eaten his full Monday breakfast and then had a snack at lunch, like nothing was wrong. And, you know what? He hasn't turned back since! That was two years ago.

What are the recommended starting doses for animals? Can you overdose an animal, and what are some common side effects?

Dosing is one of the most common questions we get, and one of the most difficult to answer. Like with people, the golden rule is "Start Low, Go Slow," but that doesn't help most people who are just starting out! How low is low? How slow is slow?

But let's look at just some of the factors that need to be considered when determining a starting dose:

1. Dose of what? Cannabis has over 100 cannabinoids and over 120 terpenes, as well as flavonoids, sterols, fatty acids, etc. Each plant and each product can have a different chemical makeup. So when people ask, "What is the dose?" the response is, "Dose of what?"

2. What is the goal of therapy? The product and dosing may be different for a patient who needs help sleeping at night, or mild pain relief vs. a patient with refractory seizures. So, before providing dosing recommendations, we need to understand what our goals of therapy are.

3. Individual factors. Some patients are naturally more sensitive to some of the adverse effects seen with Cannabis than others. They may also be on pharmaceutical drugs that can heighten or impair the effects of some cannabinoids. So, understanding the individual patient, their past response to medications, and knowing a complete list of their current medications is an important part of dosing.

The best advice is to have an open and honest discussion with your veterinarian about the use of Cannabis. If it is not an area that they are familiar with, ask them for a referral to a veterinarian that is.

Although products with little or no THC have been shown to be very well tolerated, some side effects have been reported, including sedation, changes in appetite, and diarrhea. Changes in some blood test results (alkaline phosphatase) can also occur.

Products that contain THC have a greater potential to have adverse side effects, particularly when consumed in excess, or by individuals who are particularly sensitive. When affected, animals (most commonly dogs) can exhibit incoordination, lethargy (or agitation), dilated pupils, increased sensitivity to touch, light, and sound, urinary incontinence, vomiting, and in severe cases, depressed body temperature, heart rate, respiratory rate, and even coma.

For those using products with THC, it becomes even more important to work with your veterinarian to ensure that they are being used safely and responsibly.

What changes in the industry do you foresee coming in the future?

I see more Cannabis-based pharmaceutical developments. Cannabis health products (CHPs) have been proposed in Canada which would allow the development and sale of products containing Cannabis, as well as other health products, without a prescription. These products would require both safety and efficacy studies in order to be approved and would be able to make a health claim for minor ailments (when supported by studies).

I also expect the development of custom-formulated products that use specific ratios of cannabinoids and terpenes to target specific conditions.

What do you wish people knew or understood about Cannabis?

Cannabis is a remarkable plant with the power to heal all sorts of things – not just people and animals, but the earth itself. Cannabis cleans the soil, is a rapidly growing renewable resource capable of being made into plastics, paper, textiles, and fuels, and can be a wonderful food product. It is time that we move past the stigma of the last century and begin to embrace Cannabis for what it truly is.

What is important to look for when selecting a Cannabis product for a pet?

In a perfect world, I would like all products being used for pets to have high-quality, scientific studies completed by species for the condition that is being treated. These studies should have both a safety component, as well as efficacy testing, to show that they are both safe and effective at the dosing suggested.

As it may be some time before these products are readily available, it is important for consumers to know exactly what they are purchasing. This can be more difficult than one might think. Without a regulatory body to oversee the products available on the market, what is on the label is not always what is in the bottle. So, pet families should always ask to see a laboratory analysis that shows the cannabinoid content, terpene content, as well as testing for microbes, heavy metals, solvents, and pesticides. It is also important that this testing has not just been performed, but performed on the product they are purchasing. (Not the crude ingredient, but the final product, from the same batch or lot number they have.)

In selecting a product, it is always recommended to work with a veterinarian knowledgeable in cannabinoid medicine so they can help guide product selection towards the type of product that would be most suitable.

Dr. Sarah Silcox

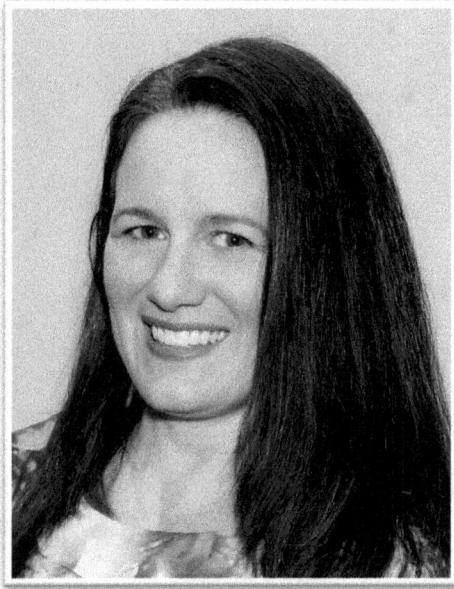

Dr. Sarah Silcox is a pioneer in the world of veterinary Cannabis use and is one of the founding directors and the current President of the Canadian Association of Veterinary Cannabinoid Medicine. A small animal veterinarian with over 20 years of clinical experience, Dr. Silcox has been active in both general and emergency practice, founded her region's first integrative medicine pet care practice, and is currently operating the region's first veterinary practice dedicated to palliative, hospice, and end-of-life care for pets.

A passionate advocate for the veterinary use of Cannabis and cannabinoid medicine, her interest in the potential benefits of medical Cannabis for pets reaches back several years. With changes in legislation surrounding Cannabis occurring around the globe, she is excited about the potential for veterinarians to begin utilizing Cannabis-based therapies in practice, and improving the quality of life of animal patients worldwide.

Stephen Cital

Describe your journey with Cannabis and your area of expertise?

My journey with Cannabis has been fraught with disdain to full acceptance. As a child, my father indulged in recreational use that gave me a negative bias (given the fact there were many other confounding circumstances at the time which included a custody battle). Like most teenagers, I was exposed to recreational use again and learned to enjoy periodic use, dampening my previously held negative bias. As an adult, I now consume Cannabis almost daily to aid in sleep quality and benefit from its general anxiolytic effects when micro-dosed.

I have found since incorporating Cannabis regularly, my professional life has been elevated. As a boarded veterinary technician specialist in research anesthesia and now industry, my days can be very challenging. Cannabis has allowed me, as a person, to be more centered by providing better sleep and pain relief for a career that can break your mind and body.

When did your interest start in Cannabis and why?

Having experience with recreational use, I started incorporating Cannabis therapy into day-to-day practice after pet owners would inquire for their terminal pet. Seeing pets were not being managed appropriately with traditional pharmaceuticals, I took the risk in condoning the utility of Cannabis molecules into the treatment of pets, despite potential legal repercussions at the time. After seeing pets thrive with the introduction of these molecules, I could no longer ignore the amazing potential and decided to expand this practice outside of terminal palliative care situations.

Not receiving formal education on the endocannabinoid system or phytocannabinoids, I decided to dedicate myself to understanding this elegant system on my own time. I became obsessed with understanding everything about the ECS and the Cannabis plant chemicals. From there, I decided to share my knowledge at veterinary conferences - having already established myself as a lecturer on anesthesia and pain management. As one can imagine, this then snowballed into conducting my own research, writing on the topic, and I am now a veterinary industry expert.

What are the misconceptions of Cannabis?

In the veterinary field, the largest misconception being perpetuated by organized veterinary medicine associations like the AVMA is that there is no research. As any Cannabis enthusiast or researcher knows, this could not be further from the truth. With over 23,000 published articles on the topic of all things relating to individual cannabinoids, the ECS and therapeutic potential in vitro and in vivo, in over 20 different species, we must stop with this misinformed understanding.

What are the questions you are most frequently asked?

The questions I am most frequently asked about Cannabis in animals are likely very similar to what one may see in the human medical field. Some of these questions include:

1. Is Cannabis safe for my pet or patient?
2. What dose should I use?
3. What studies have been done?
4. What are the side effects or possible drug interactions?
5. What product should I use?

What questions should people be asking?

When I give a Cannabis consult with a pet parent, I often try to empower them with a few questions to ask a producer or their regular veterinarian. Some of the questions I suggest they ask specific companies are:

1. Can I have a full certificate of analysis for your product before buying?
2. Has your company completed and published any studies using your product?

Questions I tell them to ask their veterinarian are:

1. What is your understanding of Cannabis use in pets?
2. Are you adverse to me utilizing Cannabis products for my pet and if so, why?
3. Have you researched this option in depth?

Give me a few examples of a positive experience, benefits, or success stories.

I really have too many to decide. I have seen animals at death's door finally able to pass comfortably and with dignity with the addition of Cannabis. I have seen geriatric dogs that spent their days pacing, sleeping, or displaying symptoms of severe cognitive dysfunction, wake up again! To the extent the owners mention their geriatric dog is acting like they did when they were a puppy. My personal dog, who has cervical disc compression, benefits from cannabinoids instead of putting him on non-steroidal anti-inflammatories.

What are the recommended starting doses for animals? Can you overdose an animal? Are there any side effects?

Dosing Cannabis products for animals is dependent on the cannabinoid profile. Like the art of anesthesia, this can be a very personal and variable strategy from practitioner to practitioner. In general, I like to dose both cats and dogs starting with a lower dose ranging from 0.5-1 mg/kg twice a day based off the total phytocannabinoids concentration derived from hemp specifically if the pet owner wants to use these products for pain, allergies, cognitive dysfunction, or other less severe ailments. For disease processes such as cancer and epilepsy, I will go much higher, doubling and even quadrupling the dose mentioned before.

For pets that I feel would benefit from higher levels of THC, I will start dosing based on the THC concentration of the product. This usually is starting the pet at 0.1 mg/kg twice a day and dose escalating to the desired effect and to build up tolerance to THC.

Give me an example for how Cannabis was life changing for someone you know.

Cannabis has been life changing for me in a few different ways. My sleep quality is better and my ability to tolerate and even medicate with Cannabis for anxiety has been incredible.

Professionally, I never thought I would end up in this industry. The growing acceptance and legalization of Cannabis has allowed me to learn new skills and, more importantly, has given the veterinary field a safe and effective alternative to pharmaceuticals.

While the correlation of how this new option is life changing, I would like to point out that healthcare professionals in general often carry an extra burden even when off the clock. We constantly worry about our patients. Knowing that Cannabis is an option now gives me the ability to worry less knowing the patient has this safe alternative option.

How has Cannabis helped you/clients/others where other products were unsuccessful?

Cannabinoids in general can be used alone or in combination with traditional medicines. In the anesthesia and pain management world, we strive to create what are called "multi-modal" protocols which means we should use multiple different medicines at lower dosages to achieve the same effect as one drug being used at a higher dose. Since we can use much lower dosages when creating these types of protocols, we can significantly decrease or even eliminate side effects. Cannabis unto itself is a multi-modal product that only adds to the quality of care we can provide our patients.

What changes in the industry do you foresee coming in the future?

I foresee more interest and research into minor cannabinoids, terpenes and flavonoids. I also foresee the discovery and processing of non-Cannabis phytocannabinoids for various conditions.

What do you wish people knew or understood about Cannabis?

Cannabis and the products you can currently buy are not all the same. A one-time attempt and benefit from this plant's medicinal potential is an experience and may require some experimentation to find a cannabinoid/terpene profile that works best for them or their pet.

What is important to look for when selecting a Cannabis product for a pet?

When choosing a product for pets, consider the following:

1. What are we trying to treat?
2. What does this profile of the product?
3. Has this product had any scientific backing with a clinical study?

4. What other adulterants might be in this product and does the company provide a certificate of analysis?
5. Do I have a veterinary Cannabis practitioner to lean on if I have questions?

Stephen Cital RVT, SRA, RLAT, VCC, VTS-LAM (Res. Anesthesia)

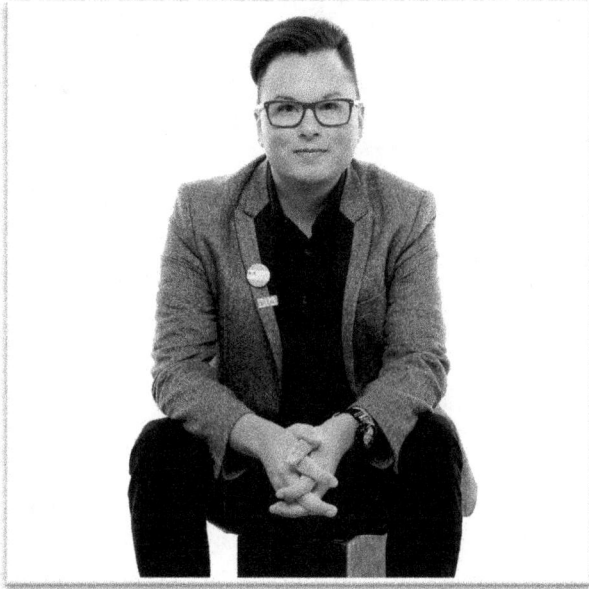

Stephen Cital is a multi-credentialed veterinary technician specialist spending the last 15 years in private, specialty practice and academia/research. He has always had a passion for anesthesia and pain management which led him into the field of cannabinoid therapy for animals. He is currently the Director of Education and Development for ElleVet Sciences where he is involved in protocol review and creation for clinical studies and education of veterinary professionals. Stephen is the co-founder for the Veterinary Cannabis Academy and research librarian for Veterinary Cannabis Education and Consulting. He is also the primary editor for a textbook focused on the use of cannabinoids in veterinary medicine being written by over 30 veterinary specialists. Stephen is the author of numerous publications on veterinary pain management, anesthesia, and Cannabis therapy for animals.

To date, Stephen has spoken on the topic to thousands of veterinarians and nursing staff at all of the major veterinary conferences such as AVMA, VMX, WVX, Fetch, etc. He has also lectured at the Cannabis Science and Technology Conference.

Christi Powell Chapman

What is your area of expertise?

I have always had an affinity for health which is why I became a nationally accredited respiratory practitioner in 1990. I've always been interested in the lungs, in particular, because of my family history.

My stepfather suffered from the effects of COPD for 12 years before passing away when I was 16 years old. My mother wanted me to follow in her footsteps and become a nurse, but I felt that I needed to make a difference up close. COPD affected me deeply because I saw how he suffered. I felt the need to alleviate that suffering for others so I chose to be a respiratory practitioner.

When did your interest in Cannabis start and why?

My interest in Cannabis began when I got ill with fibromyalgia. After several years of dealing with chronic pain, I was looking for alternatives to what the doctors had been offering. The idea of going back to school for a different career was inviting. I needed to further my education, and I needed a job that didn't require 12-hour shifts at the hospital. I started to utilize Cannabis for pain, but quickly realized I was unable to study well and smoke Cannabis at the same time. So, I went on a search for a topical and a dispensary referred me to a salve for the pain. After receiving much-needed relief, I knew my life was about to shift. My new views on Cannabis would change my life. I realized that I could function. The relief from pain changed my daily routine, which changed my thinking. I was once again engaged in life. Only this time I was free from multiple pain medications,

Gabapentin, and several other medications, which were to alleviate the side effects. Today, I get to live my best life because of
what Cannabis has done for my health. I live an active life, while
getting to work with others, improving their quality of life.

What are the misconceptions of Cannabis?

Some misconceptions about Cannabis is that it is only for
adults and that it is just used to get high. I enjoyed getting high
in my younger years; later in life, I used Cannabis medicinally
because it was what I needed for relief to get through pain issues.
Life as I knew it had changed after realizing this plant was sustaining people's lives with health and wellness. Nothing would
be the same. As a respiratory therapist, I had worked at OHSU
in Portland, Oregon. I recall working on the pediatric floor where
children with epilepsy were given sedatives for their seizures.
Sometimes such high doses were required that the patients
would need special monitoring for their breathing. Today, with
selective cannabinoids in place of so many other medications, the
quality of their lives would be so very different. Cannabis offers
that quality.

Another misconception about Cannabis is that you must be
heavily medicated in order for it to be effective. Micro-dosing
THC can bring great relief without the feeling of being heavily
sedated. CBD is effective in higher concentrations which directly
activates the 5-HT1A serotonin receptor. This protein receptor is
implicated in a range of processes, including anxiety, addiction,
appetite, sleep, pain, nausea, and vomiting. This is one reason why
metered dose inhalers became imperative for me. The ability to
get CBD in, while bypassing the gastrointestinal tract, kept nausea
and vomiting at bay.

What questions are you frequently asked on your topic?

The question I get asked most frequently is, "Does CBD get you high?" CBD is short for cannabidiol and acts very differently than its cousin THC, delta-9 or tetrahydrocannabinol. THC is psychoactive, where CBD is non-psychoactive. Research into hemp-derived CBD was made available with the 2014 Farm Bill. Research is still revealing more that this miraculous plant has to offer. Children and adults are finding a new way to live. Epilepsy has seen a vast decrease in seizures from patients using CBD. We always encourage the full plant for optimal benefits. We also recognize there are circumstances where the CBD isolate is necessary.

What questions should users be asking?

Where did it come from?

Was it third-party tested? We want everyone utilizing the safety measures that have been put into place to ensure health.

How does it affect your life? The Mind Project was one of the first to study how Cannabis affects older adults. This study found encouraging and even exciting data. They found that three months into their medical Cannabis treatment, a small group of 24 people showed significant improvement in tests of cognitive function. One thought was pain inhibits our cognitive abilities. Utilizing Cannabis can aid us in improving cognitive abilities. I'm game. There are 400 chemical compounds in Cannabis, more than 60 are known as special cannabinoids. These bond with a recently discovered system in our brain that interacts with naturally produced cannabinoids. These cannabinoids play multiple roles, affecting mood, appetite, memory, pain response, blood sugars, and much more.

Give me a few examples of a positive experience, benefits, or
success stories.

When visiting a dear friend who is a veteran, I learned that he
was taking multiple medications to relieve the pain and anxiety
and, was also suffering from PTSD. My heart sank. He was experiencing neuropathy to the point he was unable to walk or get
out of his chair at times. Currently, he is on CBD topicals and
oils. His relief has been life changing. He says his life is rich and
he can now do things he enjoys like riding on his tractor cleaning
his property, fishing in his boat with his wife and grandchildren,
and even riding his Harley again. His life is richer and fuller. I
love these two so much.

Brian Bergman, a dear friend of mine, had a wound infection
that lasted a year which nearly caused him to lose his life in the
ICU. The infection never completely cleared up and the wound
continued to open. It was so bad that he required surgery because
the wound would not heal. I spoke with the wound care nurse
and asked if we could try something new since it wasn't healing.
She agreed to let me try. As a quadriplegic, he was already compromised. Since his reserves were low, surgery needed to be his
last option. After applying high THC and CBD topicals for several
months, the wound finally closed and no surgery is required at
this time. Brian is an amazing man and has taught me many
lessons. He is always positive and is always moving his life forward. He is an owner of several dispensaries here in Oregon and
is always on the go encouraging others.

What is the recommended starting dose for clients?

I always recommend clients start low and titrate up to your
optimal dose. When do you feel the relief? That is your dose. For
THC, a good recommendation would be to start with 5 mg, wait

45 minutes for the full effect, and at that point, consider whether another 5 mg dose is desired.

Can you overdose, and what are the side effects?

Cannabis is perfectly safe to use and it carries health benefits. Overdosing on Cannabis is unlikely, if not entirely impossible.

Give an example of how Cannabis has been life changing for someone you know?

My best friend of 50+ years, Jana, is a nurse and she currently has cancer. Until now, Jana never consumed Cannabis. She is currently using gummies for sleeping and tinctures for relief from the sores resulting from the oral chemo. She is finding relief with topicals which improves her mobility and decreases the body pain associated with chemo. She has reported that life has become bearable in such difficult times.

She recently returned to work. At first, she had difficulty with endurance, but now she is experiencing more vitality and can start enjoying life again. Prior to having cancer, she was a very active, vibrant woman; she was able to do cartwheels on the beach and had been a cheerleader in high school. She is a strong woman of God and has taught me over the years what real strength is. I'm grateful to have her in my life. I love you sister.

How has Cannabis helped you or your clients where other products were unsuccessful?

Cannabis has helped me change my life. After living on a pain contract with my doctor for several years, I was finally able to find a better way for me. I was able to gain my life back with the relief Cannabis brought to me. After some time, I realized there was an underlying health issue; I really needed Cannabis even more so. I was diagnosed with a severe case of IBS; I lost so much weight my doctor became concerned and threatened to put me on medication to help me gain weight. It was at that time I started educating myself on CBD inhalers. I was at my lowest point with IBS and knew it could only get better.

One month after utilizing CBD inhalers, I gained 50 pounds to the amazement of my doctor. CBD meter-dosed inhalers allow immediate onset relief which allowed me to be hungry and eat again without constant pain and nausea.

What changes in the industry do you foresee in the future?

I foresee more people coming together for the good of healing others.

What do you wish people knew or understood about Cannabis?

One of the things I wish people understood is that Cannabis is a beautiful healing plant despite its reputation. Cannabis is a healthy alternative to taking many other medications that can be so harmful. CBD stimulates the endocannabinoid system, guiding it into homeostasis. We also know that THC has an important part in this process, as it assists in the lock and key process. There are two cannabinoid receptor types, receptor type 1 known as CBD1 and receptor type 2 (CBD2). CBD1 receptors are located in the brain, the central nervous system, intestines, connective tissue, and more. The ability cannabinoids have to activate these receptors is huge.

Activating CBD1 receptors stimulates the relief of depression, lowers intestinal inflammation, decreases leaky gut syndrome, lowers blood pressure, and anxiety. The CBD2 receptors are found in the spleen, tonsils, thymus, and mast cells, which are immune cells, monocytes, macrophages, B and T cells along with the microglia; there are smaller numbers located in the brain. Activating the CBD2 receptors induces macrophages to destroy a protein (beta-amyloid) which is a plaque found in the brains of Alzheimer's patients. When we feed our bodies the correct cannabinoids, our CBD1 and CBD2 are activated, changing how the body heals. Our bodies are intricate and have the ability to heal with nature more than we realize.

What is the difference between Isolate and Full-Spectrum?

The Cannabis plant has compounds called cannabinoids. The main ones that we have been hearing about are CBD and THC. There are hundreds more, and more are being discovered. Full-Spectrum includes the whole plant or a full profile of extracted compounds. Compounds of the plant have shown to be more effective treating disease than any one isolated component. CBD alone has healing properties just as THC does. It is when we put them together Full-Spectrum, they assist each other in doing the best job, together. This is known as the entourage effect. Isolate is CBD only (which means it does not contain THC), allowing relief for those with life circumstances that do not allow them to use a full spectrum product. CBD has anti-inflammatory properties. CBD also changes the brain's response to serotonin. Many people are fearful of THC which creates a teaching opportunity. When people know, they are able to move past fear and towards health, wellness, and wholeness.

What are the health benefits related to using Cannabis?

The health benefits related to using Cannabis are vast including helping patients with Alzheimer's, appetite loss, cancer, Crohn's disease, eating disorders, epilepsy, glaucoma, mental health, PTSD, and multiple sclerosis (adds to plasticity of MS). Research suggests that cannabinoids can reduce anxiety, inflammation, kill cancer cells, and stimulate hunger. Chronic pain is a leading cause of disability, affecting more than 25 million people.

What different effects do CBD and THC have on the respiratory system?

CBD decreases airway hyperresponsiveness in the respiratory system; also as an anti-inflammatory, this also creates bronchodilation. The collagen fiber content in the airway and alveolar sacs are also positively affected by CBD. This is promising news for the asthmatic or respiratory compromised patient. THC on the other hand, is known for inhibiting tumor growth, and killing cancer cells.

What are the effects of Cannabis on asthma, COPD, and lung cancer?

Cannabis dilates the lungs and is an anti-inflammatory. The medication given freely to asthma and COPD patients often causes tachycardia, an uncomfortable side effect not seen with inhaled cannabinoids. Several states have approved medical Cannabis for COPD treatment. CBD is also know to treat fibrosis in the lungs. There is much research to be done with what appears to have great promises in relieving respiratory distress.

Does CBD help people with lung disease?

CBD has been shown to reduce pain, help with sleep, reduce inflammation, support the immune system and reduce phlegm, and is an expectorant. These things can aid a person dealing with lung disease, as they benefit from their CBD1 and CBD2 receptors being activated. CBD has shown to shrink fibrosis in the lungs and open up airways.

How does one choose the right CBD products?

When selecting a CBD product, you should always ensure third-party testing has been done. Look at the milligrams. Is the product terpene enhanced for a better effect? Remember, applying topicals to your skin will not give you a psychoactive effect.

If you are planning to use a topical, I definitely suggest full spectrum. THC does not cross the blood brain barrier as a topical. Caution: keep away from eyes – these are for external use only.

Do you have a favorite product you use?

One of my favorite products is the metered dose inhaler. The research is very promising. It is the only immediate onset modality; heat free, and smoke free. Keeping our lungs healthy as we treat other ailments is important. My passion for helping others heal, and my own health struggles, led me to create Emerald Daze Hemp, LLC and The Balmb Body Care. Bringing reliable products to people to live healthier, richer, and deeper lives gives more purpose to living.

Christi Powell Chapman

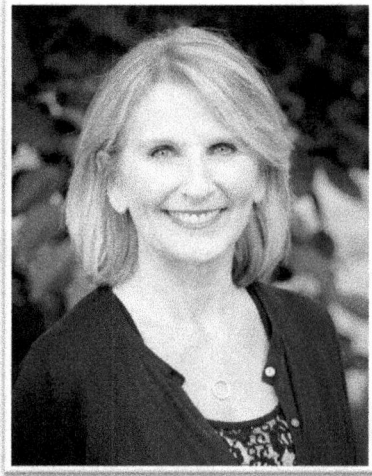

Christi Powell Chapman, a nationally accredited respiratory practitioner has worked in the Portland and Vancouver area for 26 years providing critical care and support for patients. Powell also created The Balmb Body Care in 2015, a Cannabis-based body care line. Her award-winning Balmb Body Care product line was recognized by the Dope Cup in 2016, which led her to start Emerald Daze Hemp, LLC in 2017. Emerald Daze was mentioned in *Forbes* magazine after being in the 70th Emmy Award green bags.

Barbara Blaser

Tell me about your journey with Cannabis.

I was born in a two-bed hospital on the Indiana/Kentucky border in 1945. I grew up in a small Indiana town where I graduated in a class of 18. We had three TV channels and if anyone in my town knew of, or used Cannabis, I never heard about it. Ask me about white port and Kool-Aid; that was another story.

In 1963, I attended nurse's training at a school in Chicago. When I left for school, my mom was in the driveway waving goodbye exclaiming, "Be a nurse, you will always have a job!" This was quite prophetic since it is 2019, and I am still working as a nurse.

I have been a registered nurse since 1966. Most of my professional experience has been in the mental health field. Cannabis was not really an area in which I had either a clinical or personal interest. If asked, I would say, "It's not my issue."

That was, however, until 2013. Following a "minor" medical procedure gone bad, I was left in a coma, on a ventilator, struggling to survive. Against all odds, I regained consciousness. It took six months to relearn to walk. I had a feeding tube for an entire year. I developed an allergy to morphine and codeine that caused me to lose my hair.

As I slowly recovered from this acute episode, I was left with chronic pain, anxiety, insomnia, and PTSD. I was scared and angry much of the time.

Almost overnight, Cannabis became my issue. Like many people, I was very concerned about opiates and developing a potentially deadly addiction. I began the road to both personal and clinical interest in Cannabis.

During my prolonged recovery, I did extensive research on Cannabis. There were very few mainstream classes available on the subject; certainly none at local academic venues. I did learn about a training center in Oakland called Oaksterdam University. Luckily, I was able to attend several of their classic seminars where I learned the nuances of the plant, politics, history, and legal issues surrounding the Cannabis industry. I met some of the movers and shakers in the Cannabis industry and began to understand how important the plant was to many people.

During my recovery process, I also needed to renew my nurse's license which required 30 hours of continuing education courses. I chose to only take courses on diseases that meet the qualifying conditions under the California Medical Marijuana Act. These included, but were not limited to, diseases such as anorexia, arthritis, cancer, chronic pain, HIV/AIDS, glaucoma, migraines, severe muscle spasms, and seizures.

Note – the Act also states, "Any debilitating illness where the medical use of marijuana has been deemed appropriate and has been recommended by a physician." This is a huge area that has allowed people with diseases that often mimicked the symptoms of covered conditions to legally access the healing powers of Cannabis.

Even though I was learning about Cannabis, and had access to product, I was nervous and skeptical until 2016, when I accepted a position as the Director of Clinical Services at Magnolia Wellness, a Cannabis dispensary in Oakland, CA. (Did I mention it was my daughter's dispensary?)

For the first several months at Magnolia, I conducted focus groups and met individually with medical patients who came to Magnolia. Based on what seemed to be a prevalent lack of information on the therapeutic value of Cannabis, Magnolia put together an educational program to help people understand concepts like "start low and go slow." Classes were often informal discussion groups, offering the opportunity to meet with people who might have similar medical issues.

Since 2018 and legalization, we now see both medical patients and adult recreational users who are very often interested in learning more about Cannabis. Magnolia offers training events in churches, temples, assisted living facilities, and private homes. As part of our community outreach program, I will go pretty much wherever people gather to learn principles like, start low, go slow.

As a registered nurse, I often take 3-5 appointments in a day. I work very hard to stay within the limits of my nursing license, as well as the Board of Cannabis Control rules. Every person I meet with is informed that I cannot make Cannabis recommendations. One of the first things we discuss is whether or not they have met with their personal physicians to discuss the possibility of using Cannabis. Many are concerned that their physicians may not be supportive. We seriously discuss the issue and examine the risks and benefits of having their doctor on board. For those who prefer not to contact their treating physician, they are told there are Cannabis specialists in the East Bay they may wish to meet with.

What is your area of expertise?

I am so impressed with the nurses I have met through the Cannabis Nurse Network. Many are young, bright, and enthusiastic about Cannabis. I am in awe of their energy.

If I have an expertise, it is working with seniors. I personally, at 73, lead a full dynamic life and I use Cannabis. I am almost a poster child for aging successfully. I have found that many seniors are looking for a trusted nursing professional that they can relate to. While my path to Cannabis may have been dramatic, many seniors can relate to the pain, insomnia, anxiety, and PTSD that I still suffer with.

I believe I am often acting almost as a tour guide into the world of Cannabis for new users. People need to know where to even start exploring Cannabis.

The road to successfully experiencing Cannabis, both for medical users and as an adult user, has a logical beginning and middle. Knowledge is the key to the journey.

Having a nurse as a tour guide is such a unique position to have available.

When did your interest in Cannabis start and why?

My daughter, Debby Goldsberry, has been a Cannabis activist since the 1980s, so I have always been supportive of legalization but had not tried Cannabis myself. I was superficially "interested."

However, when someone would ask about what Debby did, I would reply she worked for an alternative crop group. I remember finally telling my dad, who was raised on a tobacco farm, that Deb was trying to get Cannabis legalized. He said, "Good, farmers need an alternative crop!" Go Dad!

What are the misconceptions of Cannabis?

In the beginning of my Cannabis career, there was a widespread belief held by new consumers that you had to get high to use Cannabis, even medicinally. Many people had seen "Reefer Madness" and had negative, stereotypical beliefs about Cannabis users. Hippies. Unwashed. Prone to violence. Probably unable to hold a job. Up all night. Sleep all day. Drive high, cause wrecks. Fat from munchies. Sex in the streets.

In the beginning, new patients would often look around to be sure no one they knew saw them. Or, for sure none of their co-workers. They would speak in whispers. And, park away from the building, just in case.

Legalization in 2018, brought many changes. If it's legal, it must be ok. I worked on January 1, 2018, and I remember one of the first customers that day was a white-haired lady, dressed like she was heading to church. I was so excited. She introduced herself as being 82. I said, "Well then, you probably don't want to get high?" To which she said, "The hell I don't! None of my friends or I have ever been high and we don't want to die without trying it!"

She then asked for a pound of pot to take home for a party. I loved her. Of course, that exceeded good sense and the law. But, it was an exciting start to 2018.

On that first day of legalization, we saw complete family units that included parents who had never tried Cannabis but who, with the support of their children, were here to learn more. We saw people from cultures who had not visited us before. It was fascinating to watch the family dynamics play out as young adults tried to explain to an elderly grandparent that the crippling pain from arthritis could be relieved by Cannabis, without getting high.

That trend has continued. Seniors are looking for relief from non-addicting sources. Cannabis offers hope.

What are some frequently asked questions on your topic?

- How will I tell my family I am going to use Cannabis?
- Will this make me high?
- Can I use Cannabis if I have a heart condition?
- Will this cure my cancer?
- Can I take Cannabis to Mexico on my vacation?

These are all important questions and need to be considered seriously.

The stigma around Cannabis has been dangerous. In order for a person to use Cannabis openly, they need to get their families on board. At Magnolia, we maintain a "library" of articles that a person can take home to use for a tool in developing talking points. As more research is done, it becomes easier to engage in these conversations.

Will this make me high?

Well, maybe only if you want it to. Dosing is so critical today. In California, in a legal dispensary, things like Cannabis edibles must be packaged in containers with no more than 100 mg. Many vendors package ten 10 mg cookies per bag. Tinctures often are available from a 20:1 ratio to a 1:1 ratio. Transdermal gel pens are available in sativa, THC, CBD, and CBN so customers can decide how they want to feel. Doses may start very low – 1 drop or 1/4th of a gummy. At Magnolia, budtenders play a key role in helping customers pick the right products for their lifestyle choices. Consumers must learn to read labels. Some Cannabis products may contain more THC than a new user should be starting with.

As a medical consumer and a nurse, co-occurring medical conditions may affect the consumption of Cannabis. There are also medications that are affected by Cannabis. I take Coumadin daily because I had several blood clots during my recovery. Cannabis, for me, lengthens my bleeding time. I test my PT/INR at home and if my fingerstick gives me a reading outside the normal range, I call the anti-coagulant clinic at my hospital and they adjust my dose and tell me not to sky dive. Please check with your pharmacist for information about Cannabis interactions with any prescription medications you are currently taking.

I want to share a story. Recently, I was having tea at Magnolia with a lovely new customer who looked great but said her knees were bothering her and she wanted to try a topical. She was very concerned about possibly testing positive in a drug screening because she was recovering from a kidney transplant. If the transplant was rejected and she needed a second kidney, a positive drug test for Cannabis would kick her off the transplant list.

While topical products do not transfer into the blood, she needed to go back and talk to her doctor.

As a nurse, having read all the current information on cancer and Cannabis, I try to partner with the patients treating physical conditions. We've got you covered for nausea, pain, and anxiety. We are happy to work with your family to alleviate their fears. You want informed, well thought out discussions about treatment goals when one is making what could be life-altering choices about cancer care.

And, please don't travel with Cannabis. Not on a boat, plane, train, or car on federal highways. The laws are clear. Changing the container to an empty shampoo bottle may not save you from detection. A Tic Tac container may hold your sublingual mints but be safe. We didn't write the rules, but we recommend you follow them.

What questions people should be asking?

- How do I know if Cannabis is right for me?
- How do I decide between taking an edible, tincture, topical, concentrate?
- What should I do if I feel "too high"?
- What is a starting dose for Cannabis?
- Does it matter if my best friend prefers a certain product?
- Who should I ask for Cannabis information?

You may not know if Cannabis is right for you until you try it. Read everything you can first. Talk to people you trust about their personal experience. Consult your doctor. If you are going to try it, learn about the time it takes a product to begin working and how long it lasts. Look at your life style and your needs. Do you need something very discreet that doesn't smell?

Let me tell you how I use Cannabis for anxiety and insomnia. I take an edible and a tincture at the same time. I do low doses.

After two years, I only use the amount I need to get the relief I want. So, I do 5 mgs of a 1:1 tincture and a 5 mg THC edible. The clock starts ticking. I do the edible first. It is yummy. I want more, but common sense says, "Don't be silly. You don't want to take more than you need." It can take up to two hours before the edible starts to work but, for me, it lasts up to eight hours! Next, I put the tincture under my tongue for about 30-45 seconds. I am not fond of the taste, but it is medicine and it works, so I can do it for this length of time. The tincture starts working in less than 15 minutes and lasts two hours. So, by the time my edible is on board, my tincture is gone, I am not double dosed, and I get a good night's sleep.

Because I am old, I wake up several times during the night to use the bathroom. I am not dizzy or off balance and I can go back to sleep. I love it!

Many people, not all, are concerned about getting too high. **Start low and go slow** is so important. The "high" generally comes from a THC product. One can keep a bottle of CBD handy to combat or balance out a high. I have been reading recently that the terpenes in black pepper and lemon peel also can counteract a high. Push fluids. Rest and relax. At Magnolia, we suggest to all our customers to never try a new product on a day they have something to do or somewhere to be. We would recommend you tell someone you are trying a new product. It's better to have a plan, just in case.

A starting dose can be a drop of a tincture or half of a single square from a chocolate bar. If you buy an infused soda, pour the contents in an ice cube tray so you know just how much is in each ice cube. Use one ice cube in a glass of lemonade. Determining your own sweet spot will be your personal journey. Find the lowest dose that gives you the most relief. Don't rush. It can take several days of trying to discover the dose for you.

I love all the neighbors and friends who refer to us. Thank you all. BUT! Your dose and your preferences will need to be your own. The best piece of advice I ever got was to never eat an infused brownie made by a friend. For some people, 100 mg is a low dose. For me, that is 10 days! And don't think, "I'm a big girl, I need more." That may not be conventional wisdom. Trust me, I learned once when I mistakenly ate a large piece of banana bread with a large amount of butter! Thirteen hours later, I was still a little paranoid and confused.

Give me a few examples of a positive experience, benefits, or success stories.

I used to go to bed every night believing I might not wake up. Because of my surgery, I have to stop eating at 4:00 pm and sleep at a 45 degree angle (at least). Even if I follow all the rules, I still randomly aspirate and have had pneumonia several times.

I have trouble going to sleep and staying asleep. After much experimentation, I have found by using a combination tincture and an edible, I can go to sleep and stay asleep. If I wake up in the middle of my sleep cycle, I can repeat the tincture and go back to sleep. I do not wake up dizzy.

Give me an example of how Cannabis was life changing for someone you know.

I would like to rephrase this to "death-changing." Before I retired, I was the Director of Clinical Services at a hospice. Families and patients often experienced fear and anxiety during the dying process. While Ativan is usually available for the patient, it sometimes doesn't work. And, families seldom get any suggestions for help with that real fear and anxiety.

We see many family members seeking end-of-life relief. They have seen or heard Cannabis can help ease the transition. Often, the dying patient had previously used Cannabis.

Hospice is a service that is available for people who have a condition that is terminal but not necessarily eminent.

I worked with a lovely lady, a Holocaust survivor, who was able to leave home periodically after she starting using Cannabis for anxiety and pain. She was able to enjoy a meal out with friends. Her pain was managed, her anxiety improved, and though death came, she met it with dignity.

What changes in the industry do you see coming in the future?

- Continued improvement of products available.
- Hopefully, lower taxes.
- More choices in products.
- My big hope is we see seniors represented in the Cannabis industry. Working in dispensaries, working in sales.

What do you wish people knew or understood about Cannabis?

One size does not fit everyone. Consumers must educate themselves. **Start low and go slow**. While there is a wealth of information about Cannabis on the internet, it is not always dependable. Read books on Cannabis, read Cannabis magazines. Ask questions and write down the answers.

What are the five critical questions a person should ask before selecting a Cannabis product?

New Cannabis consumers need to be asking questions about the product.

1. What is the difference between a 20:1 and a 1:1 tincture?
2. How long does this take to work and how long does it last?
3. Can I take this if I am on a blood thinner?
4. Does this work well for treating pain? Anxiety?

5. Will I test positive if they do a random drug testing at work?

Do I really need a medical card?

This varies from state to state. Some legal states are medical only and require a medical card. In California, medical cards are not required but consumers who may need larger quantities of product due to a medical need should have the card. It also may save you money based on a dispensary's policies.

How do I choose a dispensary?

Ask the following questions:

- Do you feel safe in the parking lot?
- Is security visible?
- Is there a Cannabis smell in the parking lot? (No, please.)
- Are you welcomed in the building?
- Is the dispensary clean, neat, and well-staffed?
- Is there an adequate stock and a variety of products?
- Are the staff knowledgeable?
- Can they answer questions?

Barbara Blaser

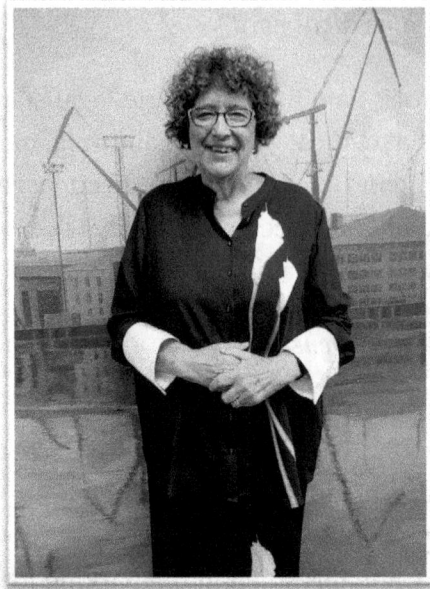

Barbara Blaser is the Director of Clinical Services at Magnolia Wellness in Oakland, CA. She works with both adult recreational and medical Cannabis clients. Barbara has been a registered nurse for over 50 years. Much of her career was in mental health and hospice. She came into the Cannabis field after a service-related medical complication left her debilitated and wheelchair bound.

Barbara says she isn't sure she wouldn't still be in that wheelchair without friends, family, and Cannabis.

Though she had retired prior to the medical disaster, she returned to work to help provide hope to people often looking to maintain their highest level of self-sufficiency.

Barbara is an author and a public speaker. She is enjoying the joy of being in her 70s and living a full and happy life.

David Wasserman

Tell me about your journey with cannabis and your area of expertise?

I was straight edge all throughout high school, meaning I didn't drink, smoke cannabis or cigarettes, or have casual sex. My parents had always told me to stay away from drugs and alcohol, and I knew deep inside that I had an addictive personality. I would consume a carton of ice cream in one sitting. I was a chronic masturbator in middle school, and I was always in trouble with the law for doing things that gave me a rush.

I tried smoking Cannabis once after graduating from high school. I contacted one of my co-workers, Matt, who didn't breathe a breath of air without some amount of cannabis, and he picked me up and packed a bong with no water in it. I had an instant panic attack and thought that I was dying. Matt dropped me off halfway between my house and halfway between the house of a girl who he wanted to hook up with. I was a little over a mile and a half from my house, and I wandered home in a slightly euphoric state. Once I got home and sat on my couch, I felt that I was in a safe space, and started to watch tv to come down. I concentrated more on the euphoria and less on the panic that was going through my body. I had no interest in smoking, and probably didn't smoke for at least two years after that.

I thought that cannabis was stupid and the kids I knew who were big potheads did nothing except smoke in the woods, and it just didn't look enticing to me.

Fast forward a few months and I was hospitalized for a bowel obstruction. My friend, Drew, came to visit me and asked me how I was doing.

306 · DAVID WASSERMAN

"They gave me Fentannnnnyl" I replied with a slur. I felt like I'd been shot in the gut, but now it's not that bad."

My mom came in the room crying. She informed me that I had a bowel obstruction and there was a surgeon standing by in case I needed surgery. "You have either Non-Hodgkin's Lymphoma or Crohn's Disease." I spent about a week in the hospital. They were able to clear the obstruction without surgical intervention. I had been introduced to opioids at this point. I learned that opioids can alleviate pain on the spot, and they can take me up to a big fluffy cloud.

I still had no interest in Cannabis. I didn't think it had a role in my life, but the role it would end up taking on in my life was bigger than I would have imagined.

During the next six months, I was hospitalized a few more times. During one stay at a local hospital, somebody told my mom, "Take your son to the University of Chicago. They are the best." I had been prescribed a variety of different medications such as Prednisone, Lialda. Entocort, and Imuran. In April of 2010, I had an ileocecectomy where doctors removed a few feet of my intestines, my ileocecal valve, and my appendix.

Soon after, a friend sent me an article on Cannabis and Crohn's Disease. "Maybe you should get yourself some edibles," Pat sent in a text following the article.

I had a small opioid habit when I started college. I had my surgery maybe five months prior, and I was going through a weird state of dissociation that lasted from a few weeks before the surgery until about four months afterward. My girlfriend in college had a penchant for smoking cannabis, but she would get so high off just a few hits that it turned me off. She would convince me to smoke every now and again, but it wasn't really my thing at the time.

During my second year of college, I had no interest in drinking. I had unfortunately taken up smoking cigarettes and that was my only social connection. My best friend, Evan, would occasionally get me to "rip a hitter with him." I started feeling the effects that other people received from smoking cannabis. Colors were brighter, everything was funnier, and knowing that we had gotten away with smoking on campus or in the dorm rooms provided even more of a rush.

From 2010 to 2015, I used opioids to cope with the pain. The same roommate who suggested that I take up lobbying as my career path told me to just smoke some weed when my disease was flaring up. "You don't need oxy, just chief on some ganj," he said. My compliance with my medication was bad, and thus my Crohn's got worse and worse. I was self-medicating with opioids because I was in so much pain all of the time. The problem was that I would just take more opioids to deal with the pain instead of actually working on treating my disease. I just wanted to mask the symptoms quickly instead of finding a long-term fix for my illness.

I discovered that pharmaceutical pills were not in abundance in rural Illinois like they had been in metropolitan Chicagoland. I noticed that while cannabis didn't get rid of the pain the same way opioids do, it would distract me from focusing on the chronic debilitating stomach pain that I felt I was unfairly forced to live with.

Using cannabis, my nausea subsided and I developed more of an appetite than I'd ever had. I applied for a medical card in 2014. I was accepted into the compassionate use of medical cannabis pilot program, but that card did more harm than it did good for me. Every time I got pulled over while driving, the officer would approach my car and ask me about my card because it would apparently pop up in bright red capital letters on their screens when checking my license. The first officer said, "I didn't even know this was a thing yet." He gave me a petty ticket and I was on my way. The next two times were similar. One officer even asked me if I was below my legal limit.

On our way to Summer Camp music festival, we got pulled over for driving 53 mph in a 50 mph zone. They found two 1/8 of weed and took everything out of the car that was packed to the brim. They went through every pocket, every zipper. I had a weekend's worth of prescribed pain medication—9 or 10 tablets I believe. If they had searched my pockets, I would have spent the weekend in jail, prescription or no prescription. The officer going through my girlfriend's car actually told her that we were essentially bringing candy to a candy store and next time to not have hula hoops visible.

The fifth time, I was not lucky. The officer called his superior officer and they didn't know the procedure. They told me to call my parents, my mom called back three minutes later, and the arresting officer said he started the paperwork. At the station, he said he wasn't going to charge me with paraphernalia, but his partner had already filed the charge.

That was my second Cannabis-related charge in only a few months.

I decided to move to Colorado. I delayed my trip a few days so that I could show up to court. I wanted to have the maximum amount of time until a warrant was issued. I was under the impression I could just wait until the statute of limitations expired. I didn't know that once you've been charged with a crime that the statute did not have an expiration date and I thought I would be okay to head back to IL after seven years. Eventually, I got everything cleared up for the low price of $3,000.

I got really sick again; I caught C. Diff and I was in an incredible amount of pain. I started using any opiates I could find on the street and then was introduced to Rick Simpson Oil. It made things a lot easier as I defeated the infection and transitioned onto a new medication called Humira. I have to inject myself every week with Humira but it gave me my life back. I stayed in Colorado Springs until 2017 and then I moved to Denver to focus on my lobbying career.

Through the maintenance medication Humira, and with Cannabis as a breakthrough medication I'm over 95% in remission. The nausea, constant out of the blue vomiting, and chronic pain all subsided. I finally found what worked for me after eight years of daily battles and struggles.

All of this, is what led me to get involved in drug policy reform. I have been studying drugs for over a decade now. I have found that the majority of harm to individuals and society is not from the drugs themselves, but as a direct result of drug prohibition.

What are the misconceptions of cannabis?

Cannabis is more dangerous than alcohol.

Alcohol is the most dangerous recreational substance. In terms of harms to both user and society Alcohol, Heroin, and Crack are the three most dangerous substances. Cannabis is actually at the bottom of the chart, with only LSD and Psilocybin-containing mushrooms (Magic Mushrooms or shrooms) being less dangerous to both the individual user and others.

Cannabis is a gateway drug.

I don't know anyone who toked on a joint before they took their first sip of alcohol. Most people who indulge in alcohol for the first time usually do so at a family gathering. Alcohol is socially acceptable and often not even looked at as a drug by many people in our society.

Cannabis is not addictive.

Any substance can be addictive. There are two types of addiction, psychological and physical dependence. While Cannabis does not cause physical dependence, it can cause psychological dependence. I think we all know someone who is psychologically dependent on Cannabis. It may not run their lives like an opioid or benzodiazepine addiction can, it can still affect their work and personal life. Addiction to caffeine is common in the United States, but it generally isn't problematic because of its availability and because it's relatively benign compared to most other addictions.

Marijuana is the correct term for the Cannabis Sativa plant.

Marijuana is a racist term that Harry Anslinger brought into common nomenclature. As the first appointed drug czar for the United States in 1930, he started a racist campaign against cannabis. He was responsible for the first national regulations of Cannabis in 1937, The Marihuana Tax Act. He used the Spanish term Marihuana and claimed that it caused people to be violent. Once the bill went into effect, statistics showed that Mexicans were nine times more likely to be arrested than white people. He was known to say racist things such as "Reefer makes darkies think they're as good as white men." He used scare-tactic statements such as "Marijuana causes white women to seek sexual relations with Negroes, entertainers, and any others." Most drug prohibition laws can actually be traced back to Anslinger. It's rumored that he actually profited off the illicit drug trade and got kickbacks from many people involved.

You can overdose on Cannabis.

One of the rumors that I have heard is that you have to smoke your body weight in Cannabis in order to overdose. The way to calculate how much of a drug is by looking up the LD50, or Lethal Dose that would kill 50% of the population. There hasn't been a verified number for Cannabis's LD50. Let's say that it was 1000mg/kg. That would mean that a 150 lb. person would need to consume 68,180 grams of Cannabis all at once. Let's face it nobody is ingesting over two ounces of pure THC at once. The cost of that alone would be astronomical. It's possible to overdose on sugar and even water. Any substance can be toxic in large enough amounts.

CBD by itself is beneficial.

Everyone's physiology is different, but what I have heard from experts in the field and medical patients who have tried every different combination of cannabinoids have told me that full spectrum is the way to go. Different cannabinoids synergize differently with one another, and by isolating individual cannabinoids you don't get the entourage effect that many patients need.

- People think that choosing a strain based off a dispensary calling it an Indica or Sativa really makes a big difference. Cannabis has been around for so long and based off breeding patterns most plants today are hybrids.
- Hemp and Cannabis are two different plants. This is not true.
- Hemp is Cannabis with a 0.3% THC content or less.
- Cannabis can make you crazy.

While it is true that some people who are genetically predisposed to have mental health issues and deal with psychosis, there haven't been any studies that show a perfectly normal person can end up in a constant state of psychosis from their cannabis use. This goes back to Harry Anslinger's propaganda. Anslinger had been known to spread such propaganda like "Marihuana is a short cut to the insane asylum. Smoke marihuana cigarettes for a month and what was once your brain will be nothing, but a storehouse of horrid specters.

What are the five questions people should be asking?

Why is the term Marijuana used instead of Cannabis?
Unfortunately, recreational cannabis use was legalized, our constitution was amended and the language that was used was Marijuana instead of Cannabis.

Where does the word Marijuana come from?
Marijuana, or Marihuana, is a Spanish term for Cannabis. Prohibitionist Harry Anslinger preferred using that term while

making wildly inaccurate racist statements about the people who used "Marihuana."

Why am I paying cash for my physician's recommendation? Also, why is a higher plant count significantly more expensive than a standard 6-plant recommendation?

Insurance providers do not currently cover the cost of medical Marijuana. A standard red card doctor will charge $80-$150 for a standard recommendation that allows a patient to grow six plants, which also means they can purchase two ounces of flower per day. Essentially, if you have an extended plant count, you can grow that many plants. I had a 75-plant count, which meant that I could grow 75 plants. I designated the dispensary a block from my house to grow my plants for me, which also meant that I could purchase 1.5 lbs. of flower from them per day.

Generally speaking, unless you are extremely ill, an extended plant count is not necessary. When my extended plant count was renewed, I was making Rick Simpson Oil which requires large amounts of flower to process. The red card doctors generally see a patient every 10-15 minutes and can make a lot of money in a single day, all cash. These doctors will charge up to $500 to recommend a plant count above 24 plants. In my opinion, it is discriminatory and takes advantage of sick patients.

Why can I be fired for using Cannabis, but not Oxycontin?

Right now, Cannabis is not prescribed. Patients receive a physician's recommendation to use Cannabis. There are very few protections in place for someone using Cannabis that has been recommended by their physician. Brandon Coats was fired from his job at Dish Network because he was using Cannabis at home, during non-working hours. The supreme court decided that medical marijuana use that is unlawful under federal law is not lawful activity and thus would not have any protection against being fired. Had Mr. Coates been prescribed Oxycodone, Dish would not have been able to fire him for his prescription use.

How can Cannabis be schedule I?

The Controlled Substances Act was created to consolidate all of the country's various drug laws using five schedules. Schedule I is the most restrictive. Substances besides Cannabis in Schedule I are Heroin, LSD, MDMA (Ecstasy), and Mescaline. Schedule I drugs cannot be prescribed and only researchers with a DEA schedule I license can legally handle them.

There are three requirements for a substance to enter Schedule I:

1. The drug or other substance has a high potential for abuse.
2. The drug or other substance has no currently accepted medical use in treatment in the United States.
3. There is a lack of accepted safety for use of the drug or other substance under medical supervision.

Schedule II is similar except there is an accepted medical use for the substance. The drug or other substance has a high potential for abuse. The drug or other substance has a currently accepted medical use in treatment in the United States or a currently accepted medical use with severe restrictions. Abuse of the drug or other substances may lead to severe psychological or physical dependence.

Schedules III-V are less restrictive and can all be prescribed by a physician and dispensed at a pharmacy. Cannabis was placed into Schedule I in the early '70s because they did not have the scientific evidence that we do today that shows the therapeutic potential for cannabis.

Give me an example for how this was life changing for someone you know.

314 · DAVID WASSERMAN

I know so many people who have benefited from this wonderful plant. Spending countless hours at the Capital for the past few years, I have seen many people use Cannabis to get off opioids or other more dangerous medications. I can tell you that many people use cannabis to treat pain, nausea, migraines, fibromyalgia, PTSD, muscle spasms, cachexia, glaucoma, HIV/AIDS, among dozens of other debilitating illnesses and conditions.

Many epileptic children find relief from having seizures by using this plant. Cannabis is an alternative to Benzodiazepines, which are one of the addicting drugs and one of the only substances that can actually kill a person from physical withdrawal. Many people think that withdrawal from opiates/opioids is bad, but you will only feel like you are actually going to die.

I always thought that Crohn's Disease was the worst thing anybody could have to deal with. Within my first few months at the State Capital, I realized that I was wrong. So many people have it worse than me.

I was in the basement of the State Capital when a child fell to the ground and started wiggling around. It all happened so fast that by the time I had realized what was happening, his mother had taken something from her purse and put it in his mouth. To this day, I'm not 100% sure if it was a lozenge or tablet or capsule, but I think it was a gummy THC or a sublingual THC/CBD edible. As quickly as the seizure started, it completely halted after she put that item in his mouth. Nobody around me batted an eye. I turned to my mentor and asked, "Did that kid just have a seizure?" He had not been paying attention, but he said, "Yeah probably."

I believe this was during one of our patient autism advocacy days at the Capital. Most of our afternoon was spent in a committee. There were multiple other children there who were struggling. I use the word struggling because as many would consider them misbehaving, I could tell that they were struggling with their existence at that moment. Maybe it was the uncomfortable benches, the boring format of a committee, their blood sugar was running low, or a number of other reasons. Whatever the diagnosis, these children couldn't sit in that room any longer. Eventually, two or three parents had to escort their children out of the big committee room. Again, this was probably something not many other people noticed, but I could sense it; I could feel their suffering.

A mother and her two children sat five or six pews in front of me. I noticed that the child to her left could not sit still. He did make it through the committee, or at least until our bill was heard. Those three hours must have been absolute torture to that child, but he made it through. This made me wonder, was this possible because of Cannabis?

I have no doubt in my mind that had he been given a commonly-prescribed benzodiazepine that morning that he could have made it through the committee, but would he really have even been there? Physically yes, but with his gaba receptors occupied, it would be the equivalent of giving his seat to a ghost.

I wanted to be a lobbyist for a pharmaceutical company, but the following day I decided that I wanted to use my communication skills to advocate for public health measures. I thought that the only way I could accomplish this would be by having one of the top pharmaceutical companies hire me as one of their lobbyists A life coach that I had hired the previous year pointed out that I was fixated on the process of getting things done. He had explained to me that there were always multiple paths to the same result. I realized that even though the path that I ended up on wasn't the path that I was trying to go down, the end result was the same.

What changes in the industry do you see coming in the future?

- Delivery of medical and recreational Cannabis
- Removal of Cannabis from Schedule I of the Controlled Substance Act
- Removal of cannabis and cannabis resin from Schedule IV of the 1961 Single Convention on Narcotic Drugs
- Veterans being allowed to have a MMJ card and own/purchase a firearm
- Interstate trade of Cannabis
- An on-the-spot test for potency/differentiate hemp and Cannabis.
- The "Amazon of Cannabis" (should be around the corner)
- The FDA will allow marketing CBD as a supplement
- Banks will work with Cannabis companies.
- Hyper-personalized administration. Technology will allow us to customize an individual's cannabis intake and the specific cannabinoids they take in based on their purported physiological benefits.

What do you wish people knew or understood about Cannabis?

Cannabis has many more cannabinoids than just THC and CBD. There are at least 113 naturally occurring cannabinoids that we have isolated from Cannabis. Each one has different effects. Each person is different, so one cannabinoid may affect one person a certain way, and have the exact opposite effect for a blood relative.

Hemp and Marijuana are the same thing. People refer to Marijuana as Cannabis Sativa or Cannabis Indica that contains more than 0.3% THC.

Cannabinoid Hyperemesis Syndrome is real. People want to say Cannabis is harmful, it's not. It's as harmless as any recreational drug goes, but no drug use is without any harm of side effects. Cannabis is still one of the safest recreational drugs in terms of harm to self and harm to others/environment. The cause of Cannabinoid Hyperemesis Syndrome is still yet to be determined. Because cannabis has been Schedule I since 1971, there haven't been many studies on it. Now that it's use is more widespread and people feel safer discussing their cannabis use with their physicians, CHS has become a widely talked about issue in the cannabis community. Some say that the increasing use of pesticides, specifically Neem Oil, may be the culprit. Hopefully more studies will be done in the future. I know of two studies scheduled to take place in the next year or so. Caffeine, one of the most widely used [legal] psychoactive substances worldwide, can give a user anxiety, insomnia, digestive issues, high blood pressure, and increased heart rate, among other things.

Cannabis prohibition has taken place in the United States since the early 1900s. Many people think that the Controlled Substances Act was the first drug control law, and they also think that Nixon was the man behind the war on drugs. The real man behind the war on drugs was Harry Anslinger.

How can we better educate the public on what is happening in the cannabis industry?

Making Cannabis less taboo is step one. When I meet people who were initially wary about Cannabis, they seem to come around when we get to the topic of legality, which is usually their main concern. Most aren't necessarily afraid of this plant because of its physical or psychoactive properties, they are afraid of it because it is a Schedule I controlled substance.

Education is key. When you walk into a dispensary, you will see advertisements for different brands and products. Many physicians that recommend Cannabis will leave a stack of business cards at the dispensaries. Also, often there will be discretionary material discussing things like potency, recommended starting dosages, and DUI penalties. "Go slow… and whatever the slogan is."

There are also organizations that the public can join or reach out to, such as my non-profit, The Southern Colorado Cannabis Council. Here in Colorado, we have several educational opportunities and locations, such as the Trichome Institute, Clover Leaf University, Inspyre, as well as approved classes from Colorado's Marijuana Enforcement Division.

In high school, we were taught about cigarettes. We also talked about drugs and alcohol at least once, but spending some time giving honest factual information about drugs, especially cannabis, alcohol, and tobacco, is necessary for children in our education system.

David Wasserman

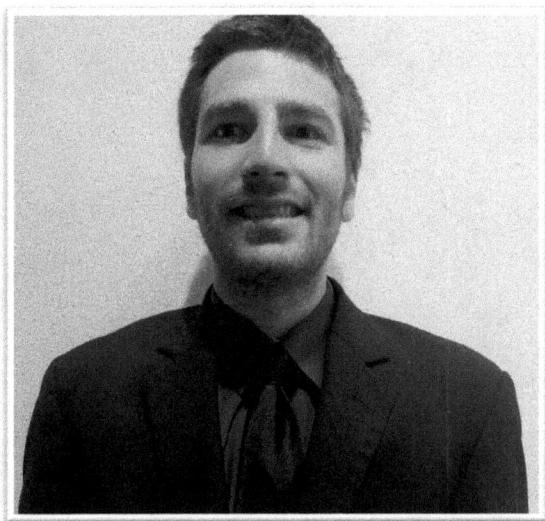

David Wasserman has been involved with in Drug Policy reform since 2015. In 2017 he took an internship with the Southern
Colorado Cannabis Council and has worked on more than 35
bills at the state capital as well as being involved in state policy
regulations. He was involved with the ballot initiative to Decriminalize Psilocybin in Denver. He volunteers with many harm
reduction organizations.

DISTRIBUTION

Kay Garcia

Tell me about your journey with Cannabis and your area of expertise?

I first became aware of the Cannabis industry when I started working at Women Grow. I am a logistics and operations expert, and I used those skills to help numerous entrepreneurs make their way into Cannabis. After five years, I've been able to extend my reach into Cannabis marketing, which is vastly different from traditional marketing. I've really enjoyed working with powerful and intelligent women to grow their businesses, and have made strong connections over the past few years.

When did your interest in Cannabis start and why?

I became interested in Cannabis when I started working in the industry. I listened to the stories people told me about their personal journey with Cannabis, and I became aware of the history behind the war on drugs. I met people who had been treated poorly by our legal system due to the color of their skin, and others who had been challenged by the medical community for participating in scientific discussions on the plant. I believe that people should have freedom of choice, and it frustrates me when policies are created that are based on falsehoods and raw emotion instead of facts.

What are the misconceptions of Cannabis?

Today, we use the word Cannabis instead of marijuana because of the negative feelings attached to the M word. Cannabis is the actual scientific name of the plant, and not a racially charged word. Cannabis is seen as cool and hip by many people, while

324 · KAY GARCIA

marijuana is seen as the tool of potheads, losers, and drug addicts. Hemp has been used for clothing, paper, building, etc. for hundreds of years, and that's also the same plant. If people realized the truth about Cannabis, and were able to look beyond the lies that have been told for the past 50 years, they'd see that you can be productive while consuming Cannabis, that it's not a gateway drug to further addiction, and that it has many benefits.

When I met the co-founder of Women Grow, before Women Grow existed, I didn't know that she smoked Cannabis daily. I worked with her and was always surprised at the work she had accomplished since I last saw her, and when I learned that she was a regular consumer of Cannabis, my entire opinion of Cannabis changed. I realized that Cannabis was not limited to the skaters behind the bleachers during high school, or the flag-waving protestors outside The White House. Cannabis was consumed by normal people way more than I realized.

What are the questions you are most frequently asked?

I'm often asked about female entrepreneurship in Cannabis, especially given the sharp uptick and current decline in female executives. I'm also asked about what type of guidance I would give to people entering the Cannabis industry, and what trends I see coming. I also offer my take to those who ask about social equity and diversity in the Cannabis space.

What questions should people be asking?

1. What can I do to promote social equity from within my company?
2. How can I encourage meaningful participation from people who have been negatively impacted by the war on drugs?
3. Who should I support in the Cannabis space - who's operating ethically and responsibly?

4. What niche should I focus my skills on?
5. What are the best resources for support and learning within the Cannabis space?

What is the recommended starting and titration dosing? Are there side effects or concerns when using Cannabis?

I recommend that people start small, especially when using edible Cannabis products. I personally use 2.5 mg of edibles and find that sufficient for me. I've had negative experiences with lesser quality products and I encourage the use of specific brands that I know undergo rigorous quality control and testing. For tinctures and topical products, when you purchase from a reputable brand, they provide guidance for their specific product. I would also recommend on your first experience (or all subsequent!) that you are in a safe, comfortable place in the company of people and/or pets that you enjoy.

Give me a few examples of a positive experience, benefits, or success stories.

A friend had an elderly aunt with tremors. We provided her with a high-quality tincture that she started small, putting just a few drops on a cracker. Within moments, the tremors ceased.

I also know of a mother suffering from hyperemesis gravidarum who used Cannabis to ensure a safe pregnancy for her child. Her child was born and suffered no ill effects (a healthy 13-year-old girl today), but the mom was fearful that her choice of medication would cause her child to be taken from her – luckily that didn't happen.

Give me an example of how Cannabis was life changing for someone you know.

I've heard lots of stories about cures for all types of ailments, or the pain relief for those with terminal conditions. I've heard remarkable experiences of entrepreneurship. I'm still amazed at my personal journey with Cannabis, though. I had no knowledge of the plant. I was not a consumer, and I was, admittedly, lost in my life and unsure of my future. When I came to the Cannabis industry, I learned a lot in a very short time, became well known due to my exposure, and my personal life changed as well. To this day, I'm consistently surprised at how welcoming this industry and the people in it can be. I was embraced and shown how to safely consume, was encouraged to share my expertise from other industries, and I was allowed time to set aside any misconceptions I had. Since my exposure to Cannabis, I've met my husband, been a CEO, traveled throughout the world learning about Cannabis, had a child, and now I'm helping other entrepreneurs find their way in this space. I cannot think of any other industry that would provide this rocket ship of a journey.

How has Cannabis helped you, clients, or others where other products were unsuccessful?

I've had personal success with minor injuries and the usage of quality Cannabis tinctures. I also have used micro-doses of Cannabis recreationally instead of consuming alcohol. Because of my position in the industry, I've heard thousands of personal stories, and many of them are rather emotional. I recall a story of a grandmother who was dying of cancer, and her Cannabis usage was part of a palliative care plan. She only had access to Cannabis flower for smoking because of her state's regulations. She was concerned about the smell clinging to her clothes, so she would not hug her grandchildren when they came to visit her. She didn't want them to know about her Cannabis usage because it has a negative stigma attached. It saddens me that these types of scenarios exist, and I make my efforts in part for the patients who cannot advocate for themselves.

What changes in the industry do you foresee coming in the future?

Banking for Cannabis companies will become a reality, with companies like Green Check Verified leading the way on compliance for Cannabis companies and the financial institutions that serve them. I see more mergers and acquisitions on the horizon, with the craft operations continuing to be successful with their niche consumer. There will be huge leaps in the medical community as clinical studies are completed, and the baby boomer generation will lead consumer spending in Cannabis products.

What do you wish people knew or understood about Cannabis?

It's not the demon that it's been made out to be. Due to the nefarious intent of a few, many have been made to suffer due to lack of knowledge or access. I've watched numerous individuals have their negative opinion swayed after a friend, family, or the individual themselves were personally touched by Cannabis. I've also seen people ascribe negative circumstances to Cannabis due to their lack of understanding. I hope that in the future, people are able to look past the emotion of the plant.

Are there any questions that you feel you would like to address that were not asked?

The Cannabis road is not an easy one, and it is not the fast money escape from the corporate world that some make it out to be. Come to Cannabis not with the expectation of fast cash, but with the idea that you have an opportunity to make a name for yourself. You can lead the way in ethical and social responsibility, and still find profits. The opportunity is here for all of us to become rich, not just in our pockets, but in our souls.

Kay Garcia

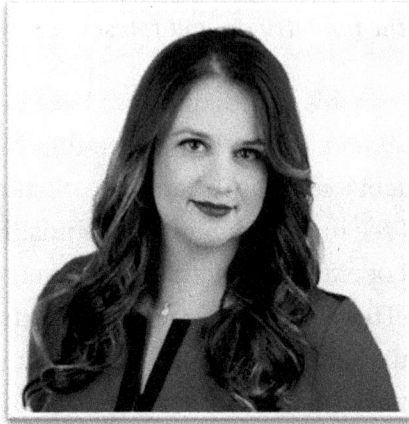

Kay Garcia (neé Neoushoff) is an expert at designing systems that enable individuals and companies to reach their full potential.

Kay began her professional career with Apple, where she learned branding, efficiency, customer service, and innovation from some of the leaders in the tech industry; an experience that fueled her desire to create simple solutions to everyday problems. She worked with Tekserve and MoviePass before joining Esteé Lauder Companies, where she led technology implementations for the company's North American Global Retail Channel.

During a year-long sabbatical from the corporate life, Kay worked as a handler on a cattle ranch, as a rural mail carrier for USPS, and as an independent consultant while living abroad in London. In 2015, Kay was recruited by Women Grow LLC, a Cannabis industry startup focused on connecting, educating, and empowering women to become leaders in the Cannabis industry. Kay was named Chief Executive Officer of Women Grow in 2017 and led the company and the nation-wide community it serves through a period of dramatic growth.

Kay currently serves on the Boards of Green Check Verified, Women's Cannabis Connection of New Jersey, and Women Grow. She is also the co-founder of Magnolia Partners.

Kay is available for one on one coaching and strategy, speaking engagements, and media appearances. Please contact for availability and rates.

Kendra K. Soderberg

Tell me about your journey with Cannabis and your area of expertise.

I've had a heck of a crazy ride with it! My journey began pre-prohibition Amendment 64 by about a decade ago. I remember the days when I had to drive 80 miles out of the way to pick up large amounts of nutrients and switch vehicles with my inner circle to avoid any potential thefts or police encounters. Being from Colorado, we had to watch our roof during the winter because the snow would melt (or large portions of it) during periods of heavy flowering; that was almost an instantaneous lead for any law enforcement officer on patrol.

The grow game is probably my top level of expertise, but I've branched out in other aspects of this industry as well.

We (my ex-husband and I) made up a team of DIY hydroponic growers to start (black market). Plants could be sold for weight, bag appeal, and smell which was our main focus at that time. We were so impressed initially (which I laugh at now) with how well we structured our system to include additional piping outside to the garden and trees; a complete closed loop which we thought was cool at the time. Everything was hidden, and it was sort of a game among our close grower network to have everything hidden, even from our closest family. Those days are long gone. I cannot believe how fast everything flipped and the industry ramped to where it is today.

I started my journey in the legit industry with a biotech company who developed blends of amendments to target different functionalities in plants. That company allowed me to travel all over the country setting up systems and implementing research trials with growers. From the west coast to the Midwest, I was very honored to move around and see different techniques, greenhouses, indoor, outdoor - the whole variance as it pertained to marijuana and hemp. Farmers were passionate. The company afforded me to expand what I already instinctually knew and more. Very exciting times indeed.

Growcentia was a very small company that started in the back of a transmission shop. I started at the very beginning, streamlining processes, mapping out conventions, registering the product in every state, and organizing our company overall. I settled into the forward-facing team, sales and hitting the market fast and furious. The beginning was super fun. We had to wash biotanks in the back and get them ready for the next batch. I'm almost positive people walking by thought we were cooking meth in there. We had a small team, young, energetic, and we had fun building that company.

The founders were a group of Ph.D.'s out of CSU who weren't even really looking into Cannabis. The bulk of their focus and trials were in farming. Another Cannabis grower, Mike Walsh, and myself, advocated heavily for Cannabis during those initial planning phases. The company had five people developing the business and several others who were linked to the university doing trials to bring that product to market. When I say this company was a startup, it was such a startup that I nearly gave myself to it for the first year, for free. The wage was laughable, but I hung in there.

We grew that company nationwide and eventually went international within the first year and half. I did a lot of heavy lifting for that organization. The headaches became more frequent as we grew, and we grew fast. I had many negotiations on my worth for that organization, but realized that when they went public, there would be no room for me and my growth, so I knew it was time to exit. I didn't look back, and I went full fledge into marijuana. I did everything from selling soil and lights, to brokering trim, flower, cartridges, writing SOPs; helping MIP's, dispensaries, and grow facilities. I started my own consulting company and worked alongside other well-known companies. I learned very quickly how ruthless it was out there. Many colleagues were acquiring funding and getting into partnerships.

I witnessed the craziest, saddest, and most profitable swings all around me. The emotions that people were experiencing in this industry were like no other that I had previously been in, and I've been a contracting geologist drilling for oil. The ups and downs are all a part of it. There were huge scams in Colorado involving powerful people. Unfortunately, I found myself in the middle of one of them at one point.

This industry can be very cruel at times, especially to women. Some have had wild success and support, but some have not and are no longer with us. We, here in the Colorado Cannabis community, are like family, so when you lose one of your own, it has a rippling effect. It was heartfelt, and the outpouring of support for our friend and colleague still resurfaces today. That was a pivotal point in my career where I switched gears out of marijuana and began focusing on hemp.

I actively started visiting farms, setting up deals, rekindling relationships, keeping a pulse on rules and regulations; so much excitement as the farm bill was inching closer and closer each day. It was invigorating knowing the movement was going forward. Farming/growing, processing, labs, products, and of course, the network – each aspect experiencing growing pains like no other because, largely, the industry as a whole is still very unregulated. I was very active in keeping a pulse on the players, the market, and local governing bodies and their affiliates.

I eventually landed a gig setting up a 73,000 sq. ft lab and processing facility. I came on as a project manager working with a fabrication team in Santa Rosa process biomass straight to distillate on an unprecedented scale. The vision was big and unproven, but we began work immediately to implement and scale. We had massive deadlines with general contractors, electricians, plumbers, engineers, and of course, staff.

The fabrication company did an overall restructuring which affected our timelines. We did come online, just not at the expected capacity, and the focus switched gears. We then began producing a well-filtered winterized crude which then was kicked downstream to several companies moving fast in the T-free, broad spectrum and water soluble/nano realms. I definitely learned a lot with this company and it gave me ammo to charge into the projects that I have my time vested in today. I have launched my own online sales marketplace, Biologic Hemp, which has strategic partnerships with several companies. We are a complete hemp supply chain management CBD + Hemp wholesale and retail.

When did your interest in Cannabis start and why?

In 1999, some friends who I snowboarded with showed me that I could pay for tickets to concerts with premium-grown bud, at prominent concert venues in Denver. It was a connector of sorts.

What are the misconceptions of Cannabis?

That it is a one size fits all. It is not. It is a tremendous medicine that works across a large number of ailments, but sometimes it's not the best option for others. More trials are needed; the numbers don't lie. I advocate for the science above all. If my grandma had a cancer where she would consume Cannabis in conjunction with her chemo and the researched shows that it works well, then I would want that for her. If my daughter had some kind of disease that proved to have some sort of drug that had outperformed any Cannabis product, then I would advocate for that for her. It doesn't have to be complicated, and I am research driven.

What questions should people be asking?

I believe industry people should be asking more about techniques and processes when it involves processing plants into a number of different verticals destined for consumption. It's a double-edge sword because a lot of the intel remains internal due to proprietary standard operating procedures. If a company has diligence, it will promote its process, without giving away intel. We know from the nutraceutical world that key words tend to become marketing buzz and we have no real idea how that product was manipulated into its final form. Testing is evolving to add to our level of comforts around these questions, but I don't believe it's foolproof yet. Companies should be honest in revealing if the product contains isolate, distillate, crude, and what stages those are at.

Where did the product come from (Growing region? Farm?) Can you prove it?

Some organizations will have a track and trace system implemented that is organized with all the proper documentation of chain of custody.

Consumers should be asking:

Have you ever bought this product before? Have you bought biomass before? Have you bought isolate before? Have you bought gummies before? What was your experience?

What is the recommended starting and titration dosing?

Start with a small (5-10 mg) dose over a six-hour period to see how it works in the system, and then you can increase from there.

Give me an example for how Cannabis was life-changing for someone you know.

A dear friend of mine, who virtually paralleled my life, and who I consider a major support system in my life, was told she had Stage 3, going into Stage 4, cancer. It was a heartbreaking moment where time seemed to stand still. She had two small girls who had recently lost their father to suicide. We scrambled to learn more and provide support to our dear friend. Since I was already in the industry, I had been watching brands and trialing some CBD products. It was the beginning of her battle and she was desperate to live for her kids.

We started with a 500 mg tincture, full spectrum Blue Bird botanicals.

She also had a vape pen she pulled on three times a day.

That was four years ago. She is now cancer free.

How has Cannabis helped you, clients, others where other products were unsuccessful?

I didn't have a major health crisis or debilitating ailment, but I was rather astounded by the results. I have three boys, and juggling work and family causes a great deal of stress. I suffered from a pretty bad case of adult acne with super sensitive skin that nothing, and I mean absolutely nothing, would help (you can name all the top acne products – tried, spent thousands on - never worked). I was already in the industry but had never used a topical crème with any consistency in my daily routine. I was given an organic topical by some local friends of mine who own a farmer collective that was one of the very first USDA certified organic hemp farms in Colorado. This stuff was so miraculous that within the first week and a half, the acne disappeared completely. I still had scarring that I had to deal with, but it was incredible to see this product work so fast in clearing up what was a visible representation of the ups and downs I had endured in a short course of my life.

What changes in the industry do you foresee coming in the future?

I already see the moves that Big Tobacco and Pharma are posturing for. It is going to be a race to the bottom just like we saw in marijuana. Companies that get in on clinical trials and pump out white papers while developing strong marketing campaigns will definitely survive.

What do you wish people knew or understood about Cannabis?

That it is the real-life conspiracy theory exposed. Cannabis was demonized and locked away while the underground, thriving black market existed, with a wide range of quality issues pertaining to product formulations and enterprise/relationship building to provide the necessary treatments and medicine to the larger underground network.

Are there any questions that you feel you would like to address that were not asked?

I would like to make a general comment to give props to breeders and growers alike who have been doing this for generations. These are the people who kept the genetics alive. They took many risks and experienced many failures to create the legacy they created. Many have moved on and are no longer fighting to stay afloat in these ever-dynamic markets; others have had their IP poached only to end up in the hands of a venture capitalist or other parties who didn't credit their work. They did more than anyone will ever know.

Kendra Soderberg

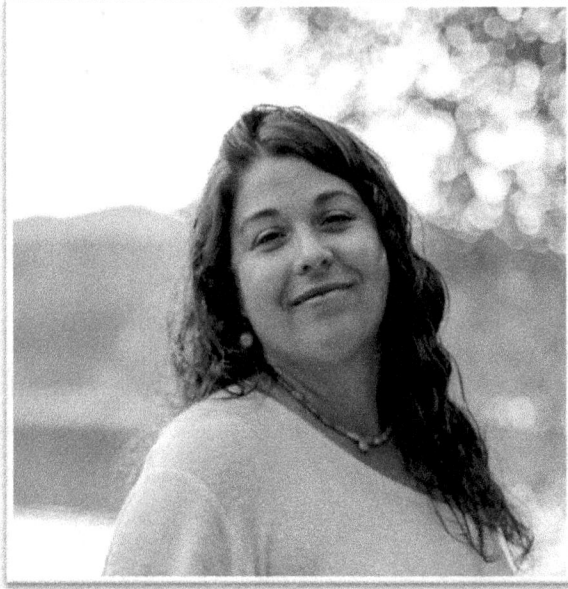

2001- 2016 Growing/ Cultivation experience.

2014-2017 Built Biotech company from small startup, implementation of new grow methodologies across the states and internationally.

2017-2018 Consulting with investor relations with MIP in Colorado, highs and lows of investor entanglement and an underfunded mismanaged marijuana infused kitchen.

2018 Current - Now consulting/contract work structuring and compliance around manufacturing, processing, grow facilities in CO (operations and production of various hemp products).

2018 Online sales (wholesale, retail, trade - hemp products)

Cannabis Professional; Over a decade of experience

Start Ups | Grow/ Ag. Operations IP | Manufacturing | Restructuring and Reorganizations | Market and Growth Analysis | Consulting | IT Integrations | CGMP | Compliance Implementation | Quality Assurance/ PCQI Certified | Network & Business IP

Total Hemp Supply Chain Management

- Online store
- Wholesale and retail
- SCO, workflow automations, inventory management
- Legal framework
- Strategic partnerships
- Manufacturing buildout coordination with GM/ contractors/ city permits department/ engineers/ staff
- Design and implement cGMP protocols and standards (SOPs)
- Quality control and assurance
- Product formulations
- Create and manage track and trace systems
- Hire and train staff
- HR implementation/integration plan
- Design and implement parameters for large scale extractions of all types

Kevin Altamura

Tell me about your journey with Cannabis; what is your area of expertise?

My journey in Cannabis began when I started studying biology and chemistry in college. My major required I take several botany and pharmacology classes. Throughout my coursework, I learned about the physical anatomy of Cannabis plants as well as the chemical properties they produce. Fast forward a few years out of college, I find myself working as a bar consultant. Part of that job consists of coming up with interesting beverage programs, some of which were Cannabis-based. My area of expertise is creating alcoholic and non-alcoholic infused beverages, and I challenged myself to create some delicious cocktails infused with Cannabis.

When did your interest start in Cannabis and why?

In college, I was able to take several medical courses. I learned how limited we were when it came to pain medications and the serious side effects associated with them. The usual pain management route is to prescribe some sort of opioid and hope that does the trick. Due to their highly addictive properties, they end up doing more harm than good. When I learned about the medical properties in Cannabis and how many patients were reporting positive outcomes, I was instantly intrigued. Since today's most common pain medications are derived from the poppy plant, it became a no-brainer as to why the Cannabis plant could possibly provide the same level of relief, or even better, without any adverse side effects. With over 110 different cannabinoids, it's only a matter of time until scientists start creating medications from these compounds.

What are the misconceptions of Cannabis?

Some of the most common misconceptions are that Cannabis use will eventually lead them to use other drugs. Cannabis is routinely called a gateway drug; but in fact, there is no evidence to support this. On the contrary, many patients in states where medical use is allowed, are using Cannabis as a direct replacement for opioids. There is also the misconception that you can overdose. To date, there has not been a verified death caused by an overdose. Scientists have proven you would need to consume well over 600 kg in a span of 15 minutes to overdose on Cannabis, which is pretty much impossible.

Give me a few examples of a positive experience, benefits, or success stories.

Edward, a close family friend, was diagnosed with advanced Parkinson's disease. After a couple years of treatments, his condition rapidly started to deteriorate. Daily tasks such as changing the TV channel were impossible. He began experimenting with Cannabis after a doctor recommended he give it a try. Since the idea of smoking was not attractive, he opted for tinctures instead. Within a week, the shaking greatly subsided! Pain levels dropped; something the prescription meds could not achieve. After five years of being introduced to Cannabis, he says he can't imagine living without it.

What changes in the industry do you foresee coming in the future?

It is only a matter of time until Cannabis becomes legal at the federal level. Once this is achieved, large pharmaceutical companies will start investing in Cannabis and start creating exciting new medications that will cater to a wide range of illnesses.

Laboratories will start engineering custom strains that will be specifically designed to alleviate specific diseases. I also see the consumption of flower being replaced with concentrates, edibles, and infused beverages.

What do you wish people knew or understood about Cannabis?

The one thing I wish people knew was the amount of potential this plant has. Currently, there are thousands of strains that have worked in treating different ailments. There is still a lot of unknown but getting the general public to understand this will only expedite the process.

Also, I would like people to know there are non-psychoactive alternatives available, which still provide medical benefits without getting you high. This should be attractive to new patients who may not want any of the inebriating effects that come with THC.

What is important to look for when selecting a Cannabis product?

Quality! That is by far the most important thing to look for when selecting any Cannabis product. Unfortunately, due to the high demand, there are plenty of producers cutting corners and selling low-grade products. Some of these products may even cause adverse health effects.

When purchasing flowers, you will have to decide between indica and sativa. Indica great for pain and sleeping disorders and is usually described as a body high. Sativa is great for mood disorders, is uplifting, and normally used throughout the day. Or, you can opt for a hybrid, which contain the best of both.

The next thing to look for is their potency, which is measured in a percentage. It is of utmost importance to pay attention to this since THC levels have greatly increased over the past couple of years and continue to do so. Anything under 10% will be considered mild and great for first time users. For the most common strains, you will be in the 11-19% range. Ease your way into anything over 20%.

Also, find out how the flowers were grown and harvested. Many producers use harsh chemicals to speed up production and increase yields and potency. The problem arises when the plants are not properly flushed, and trace metals are left in the flower. Ultimately, the consumer will ingest this, resulting in an awful taste and also, a potential health hazard arising. To avoid this issue, purchase organically grown flowers.

When choosing concentrates, be aware of their increased potency. Some can be well over 90% THC! Similar criteria apply when selecting a concentrate. First, ask how the product was made. Certain concentrates are made using solvents such as butane. I would recommend opting for Co2 extracted concentrates since they will provide a cleaner and more refined product.

Can you explain how to mix Cannabis and alcohol? What are the potential problems mixing alcohol with Cannabis? Are there recipe books that you can use or recommend? Are there certain recipes that are easier to start this process?

Infusing spirits

Cannabis, when mixed with alcohol, can make some great cocktails. When starting, it's best to begin with low dosages since it may take approximately 30 minutes to two hours to feel its effects. Do not drink more than one infused cocktail per hour since the effects will linger for several hours.

The recommended starting dosage is 10-15 mg. When ingesting Cannabis, be aware that the effects will be substantially stronger than when smoking. The liver will completely metabolize THC and convert it to be readily absorbed by the body resulting in a much stronger high.

Alcohol acts as a non-polar solvent, so it will easily dissolve any cannabinoids. To start, you must first decarboxylate the flower so it can be ingested and retain its effects. To do this, simply warm your oven to 275° F. Next, place your grinded flower onto a sheet pan. Bake for approximately 20-30 minutes. Make sure the flower does not start to burn! This process will convert THCA into its ingestible psychoactive form of THC. After decarboxylating the flower, we can begin the infusion. Pick your favorite spirit. I would recommend a Navy strength gin or an over proof bourbon such as Old Forester. Do not use low alcohol by volume spirits since it will take longer and not fully dissolve the cannabinoids. Mix 750 ml of spirit per 7 grams of flower in a non-reactive container. Set up a double boiler and place the container on top. Make sure the temperature does not exceed 170°F. Let it sit for an hour, stirring occasionally. Strain out the flower and rebottle. You are now set up to make infused cocktails.

The only downside to this method is the cannabinoid concentration will remain the same. If you would like to control your dosage, using tinctures or bitters would be the way to go – these are readily available at local dispensaries. If you would like to make your own concoction, see the recipe below.

Tincture Oil Recipe

Materials needed:

- Flower- 14 g
- Everclear (190 pf preferred)
- Rice cooker
- Coffee filter
- Mason jar

Making a tincture is very similar to the process described above. Tinctures will give you the option to alter the dosage when making the cocktails. To make your tincture, first decaboxylate the flower. Next, place 14 grams of flower with 250 ml of 190 proof Everclear into a non-reactive container. Muddle the mixture until its uniform. Let it sit for 6-8 hours stirring occasionally. Strain the mixture through a coffee filter and discard the solids. Set the rice cooker on high and pour the mixture into it. Make sure you are in a well-ventilated area! Also, ensure no open flames are near the mixture. Once the alcohol is mostly evaporated, transfer the mixture into a small mason jar or a vial with a dropper.

Cocktail Recipes

Now comes the fun part! Listed below are some of my signature infused recipes. For additional cocktail recipes, I would recommend "The Craft of the Cocktail" written by Dale DeGroff. To make these cocktails, you will need a shaker tin, Hawthorne strainer, and a bar spoon. To make the best possible cocktail, avoid using party ice since it will over dilute the drinks. Feel free to experiment and try alternative spirits and modifiers, after all, bartending is about having fun.

Last Breath

.75 oz Infused Gabriel Boudier saffron gin
(If using a tincture start with 10 mg)
.75 oz Fresh lemon juice
.75 oz Pamplemousse liqueur
.75 oz Yellow Chartreuse

Shake ingredients for 10-15 seconds. Pour into a martini glass and garnish with a grapefruit slice.

El Chapo

2 oz Infused Reposado tequila (If using a tincture start with 10 mg)
1 oz Fresh pineapple juice
1 oz Lime
1 oz Simple syrup
2 Dashes Hellfire bitters

Shake ingredients for 10-15 seconds. Pour into a rocks glass and garnish with a pineapple wedge.

Pa La Playa

1.5 oz Infused vodka (If using a tincture start with 10 mg)
.75 oz Lemon
3 Strawberries
.5 oz St. Germain
.25 oz Simple syrup
Top with sparkling wine

Muddle strawberries; shake remaining ingredients for 10-15 seconds. Pour into a wine glass and top with sparkling wine.

Improved Carre

1 oz Infused Anejo rum (substitute for 3.5 ml tincture)
1 oz Rye whiskey
1 oz PX sherry
.25 oz Benedictine
2 Dashes of Angostura and Peychaud bitters

Place all ingredients into a mixing glass and stir for 15-20 seconds. Pour into a rocks glass.

Kevin Altamura

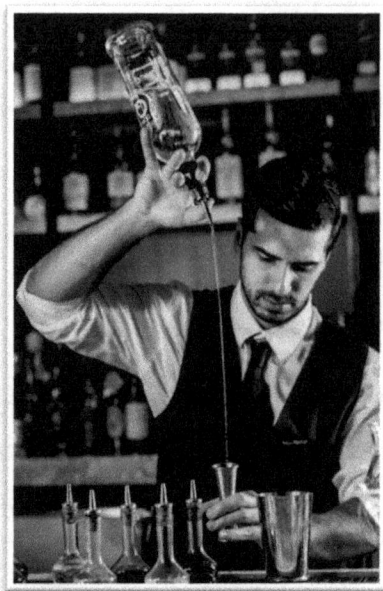

Kevin Altamura was born in Miami, Florida. He is currently working as a consultant creating new bar concepts. Over the last 10 years working in the hospitality industry, Kevin has worked in some of the most demanding bars. He graduated from Florida International University with a degree in biology.

Parisa Mansouri-Rad

Tell me about your area of expertise with Cannabis?

Marketing and branding, events, advocacy, and parenting and Cannabis.

When did your interest in Cannabis start and why?

My child was diagnosed with a life-threatening condition caused by opioids and I was desperate to find natural, less harmful relief for her. And, prolong her life.

What are the misconceptions of Cannabis?

Many people believe that when someone is high, they are out of control. Cannabis makes my child happier, and less dependent on pharmaceuticals, like anti-anxiety meds and anti-depressants.

What are the five questions you are most frequently asked?

1. Do you let your daughter smoke Cannabis?
2. Does your daughter get high?
3. Are you scared your children will be taken away?
4. What's the most effective method of consumption?
5. Why not try options that are less harmful to the growing brain?
6. Why not use CBD?

What questions should people be asking?

1. What conditions qualify a person for a medical Cannabis card?
2. What resources are available for parents and caregivers?

3. What's the most effective way to treat several conditions?
4. Should we start with CBD, and if so, what brands are trustworthy?
5. How do we safeguard against fake or misleading labels on CBD products?
6. How do we address Cannabis use with our support system?

What is the recommended starting and titration dosing?

I always recommend starting small (5 mg) and using CBD only at first. Using a quality CBD can help many conditions before even investing in a medical marijuana card.

Give me a few examples of a positive experience, benefits, or success stories.

Cannabis has improved my daughter's health. She no longer takes 15 pharmaceuticals. She's able to live and function more normally, and she can even tolerate to eat by mouth on some lucky occasions. Her nausea is so intense that, without Cannabis, she is dry heaving around the clock. Cannabis allows her to live without as much pain and discomfort.

Give me an example of how Cannabis was life changing for someone you know.

My daughter, Yazy, was on her deathbed (literally) prior to using Cannabis. I truly believe the plan is improving her current quality of life and aiding in sustaining it longer.

How has Cannabis helped you/clients/others where other products were unsuccessful?

Their pharmaceuticals nearly killed my daughter. She was on feedings tubes and IVs, and after months of unsuccessful in-patient treatment, we were sent home for palliative care. We were told to make her comfortable. We did that, and now she can walk again, eat some foods by mouth, and laughs and enjoy her time with us.

What changes in the industry do you foresee coming in the future?

I foresee federal legalization, more safeguards for patients, and more testing.

What do you wish people knew or understood about Cannabis?

That's it's a SAFER alternative to MANY pharmaceuticals we give our loved ones without even thinking twice.

About Parisa Mansouri-Rad

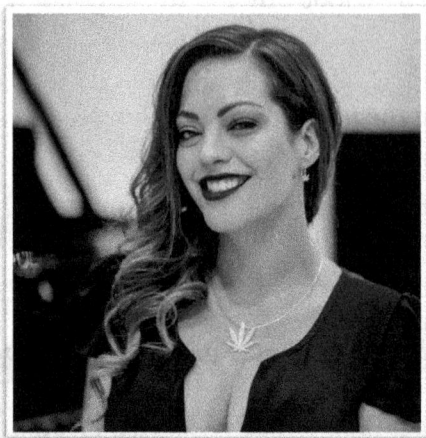

Parisa Mansouri-Rad, also known as, "The Marijuana Momma," is a marketing executive and Cannabis advocate whose experience as the mom of a special needs child propelled her into the industry. When spinal fusion surgery to correct scoliosis left her then 15-year-old daughter with a rare, life-threatening condition characterized by chronic abdominal pain, Parisa's search for palliatives led her to Cannabis (medicinal marijuana).

After witnessing her daughter's dramatic improvement, Parisa decided to leverage her marketing experience to re-brand the maligned Cannabis industry through ongoing advocacy and education of the public on the benefits of medicinal marijuana.

Parisa graduated with honors from New Mexico State University with a major in agriculture business and a minor in marketing. She serves as Market Leader Program Director for Women Grow & President of MjMomma Consulting LLC, a Cannabis focused marketing agency.

Shira Adler

"Hello. My name is Shira Adler,
and I am a recovering, formerly anti-pot parent."

This sentiment is met with a few laughs and a fair amount of quizzical looks across a wide range of audiences. I also admit to having nearly as many hashtags as I do roles and responsibilities in the Cannabis industry—and wouldn't have it any other way.

#MarijuanaMama (Reuters)
#ThePotMom (HuffPost),
#CannaFairyGodmother (Vireo Health).

Whatever you wish to call me, the purpose is the same. I'm here in service to uplift, educate, and create. So, with whomever I come into conscious contact, I am, in that moment, one of them, seeking to create a bigger circle of "us".

If I can invite people into what I call the canna-curious conversation, then I'm succeeding in my small way to help break stigma, and through my book and products, offer healthier natural alternatives to our sick care industry. My goal is simple: invite and encourage people to become their own best advocates; consumers, practitioners, policy makers, change makers—we can and deserve to live a life of vibrant wellness on a mind-body-spirit level.

That's where I see Cannabis/hemp being our best chance to do just that.

Yet for most people (still) in this country, there is a long road to go based on the staggering mountain of stigma and misinformation. To climb that mountain and break it down into a molehill is my purpose. Products to support people is one way. But there has to be a deeper conversation happening at the same time.

With every customer or person I meet when I speak at events, I share my mission by admitting that you don't know what you don't know...and there is room to grow. So, I speak my truth and humbly share my story before myriad audiences whether I am:

#ThePotMom — a marijuana activist at press conferences for proposed new legalization legislation.

At "how-to-warn-your-kid-about-vaping" PTO meetings—where I educate that it's not the vaping that's the issue, it's the devices, substances, and need to self-medicate, that are the problems.

At Cannabis and hemp conferences where I've spoken about topics ranging from the history of hemp, to social justice, to the mind-body-spirit benefits of plant-based medicine.

When sitting on FemPowered hemp and Cannabis panels where I've been flanked by equally amazing and inspiring fellow female founders, CEOs, or other C-suite members.

I repeat my opening statement as if I were in an AA meeting because it encapsulates who I've been and who I am yet becoming.

As a single, self-employed mom, I have always believed in authentically admitting to my kids when I'm wrong about something.

I was wrong about Cannabis. Many of us GenXers were because we were the first generation born from baby boomers — all of us still caught in the lingering haze of reefer madness.

There is no judgment in the statement, but rather a tie that binds... regardless of the state (or country) in which I may be speaking, the demographic of the audience, or any "surface" factors including geography, socio-economic demographic, educational, background, or belief system... or even with the team that supports my company... this much is true.

We are sharing a journey of seeking something to make our lives "better, safer, stronger." When I open my talks with a simple sentence about having been on the "other" side, it resonates. That's how we find common ground from which we can be open-minded, and open-hearted when it comes to the incredible benefits of Cannabis on a personal, familial, communal, societal, and planetary level.

Instead of starting from a place of separateness, I am seeking connection. Regardless of who we are, where we've come from, what our background or belief system, we all have certain need states. Working with our natural environments has always been how humankind has survived... and thrived. Now it's time to take plant-medicine to a higher level.

This is why I am in this industry.

I understand the concerns. I used to carry them myself and ESPECIALLY as a parent... we have fears fed by decades of falsities.

"THC is as bad as CBD."

If you can believe it, that sentence, was uttered by an actual drug counselor at a residential treatment center and boarding school for boys in upstate NY. I know this for a fact because my son was in that center at the time this nonsense was stated.

It was my son, actually, who inspired me to finish writing my book because of that statement. He was 14 at the time and stood up to correct the counselor. My son accurately discussed the neuroscience and physiological responses to his group. He explained how every mammal is wired with an endocannabinoid receptor system. He talked to them about how cannabinoids bind to those receptors like opiates to opiate receptors in the brain do, but WITHOUT any negative effects. In fact, the ERS (endocannabinoid receptor system) regulates all of your other systems, bringing the body into homeostasis.

Did I mention he was 14 when he knew all of this?

And yes, it's a dubious honor — having a kid in residential treatment for over-smoking marijuana as a minor — yet knowing that our life together, and as his mother, I had learned enough to educate not just myself, but my son. Now HE was in a place of being a teacher.

Don't get me wrong. Fighting the "system" is difficult and not for the faint of heart. However, I am not exactly shy and retiring, if you hadn't guessed as much. I removed my son from that ridiculous program, published my book, and worked with a proper Cannabis practitioner who specializes in pediatrics and teens.

My son is only one of my success stories. My daughter was also a minor when I got her a medical marijuana card and I am now a proud caretaker-card carrying member of the Cannabis fan club.

Since those days, I have gone on to work with so many families and individuals both personally, as a spiritual counselor, and through my holistic regimen and products.

Even if you're not familiar with aromatherapy, what it does, or how it's been around since the beginning of time as an ancient healing modality... the reasons for using natural products like mine are the same regardless of what you know, or where you've come from. We all have our stories... and our healing journeys.

These stories that are so different from each other — yet share striking similarities. People don't want to hurt as deeply as they have been hurting. They don't want to be dependent on Big Pharma — an abysmally failed experiment! We've never before been as overmedicated and underserved as we are in society today. People are sick, and sick of that system.

Sure, they're afraid... of getting "high," of losing their jobs — or worse — their kids, for trying a product, thinking CBD is the same as THC. Yet they're also sick of being sick.

We are now in a state of change — seeking something old that is new again.

Cannabis.

Science may want to refer to the species by the sum of its parts: terpenes, cannabinoids, flavinoids, plant enzymes... however you break it down, the end result is the same.

We share this planet with plants here to support our natural bodies and synergistically benefit each other.

I take that as a sacred spiritual contract. This philosophy informs my product development and my personal mission in connecting with people.

Ultimately, my higher goal is to remind everyone that we are not human beings trying to become more spiritual, but in fact we are spiritual beings having a (sometimes really painful) human experience.

Through that lens we have more in common than that which divides us and our synergistic relationships can, and will, improve if we create what I call "modern alchemy" — the merging of ancient plant wisdom with modern science.

This is why I started my company. I wanted not just to help my own kids (which I did) get off of Western medicine for their "special needs" — but to help others evaluate their choices, and consider options through holistic hemp, and candidly address-ing misconceptions around Cannabis.

I'm also not trying to convince anyone of anything... just sharing my story... an ongoing journey.

This is my truth — and one of the biggest issues we, in this industry face today.

Stigma. I get it.

I was anti-pot — so much so, I divorced a husband many moons ago who was a total pot-head and lied to me about it. Well, to be fair, I divorced him because the bigger issue was his lack of respect for me, not his use of the plant. After all, a spouse who hides a habit (of any kind) may not be the best partner long-term. (For the rest of that story, you'll have to read my next book *Pink Moccasins: And Other Footwear Inspired Tales Of FemPowerment*.)

Yet, the truth remains... whether or not we all come from a place of comfort and openness in consuming, supporting, creat-ing, or educating about Cannabis and Cannabis products... we all have our own histories, impressions, and experiences.

Mine was that I was hardcore anti-pot and the only times I'd tried it in high school was because of the "bad boy" I dated. I can see you rolling your eyes now... but you know you probably had one of those, too...

Anyway, aside from the minor dabbling when I was young and impressionable, I held onto those convictions by and large until YEARS later when my son (then a 4th grader) said to me, "Mama, I don't like taking those pills. They don't let me feel like myself."

Ironically, he said this to me totally unscripted, sitting on the front stoop of our home while being filmed for what was going to become the debut episode of Bravo TV's "Extreme Guide to Parenting."

So yes, on top of all that I've already shared, it's also true... I was a debut reality TV mom. In other words, I play myself on TV.

However, all kidding aside, I don't know if you have anyone in your life who has been on medication for things like anxiety, depression, ADHD, PTSD, or anything else... but I did.

I grew up with my late mother, struggling for most of my life with mental health challenges. And then gave birth to two children, who, carried diagnoses through no fault of their own (or even genetics), but because of a severe amount of trauma the three of us endured by their biological father, with whom we have had zero contact, since my second child was a newborn.

It wasn't easy.

I struggled — hard — as a single, self-employed mom and back then, clergy. I helped spiritually take care of my congregants and their families while trying to balance my own, and not just survive, but THRIVE. I wanted to make the healthiest choices on behalf of my kids and myself and sometimes that meant diving pretty deeply down into rabbit holes to leave no stone unturned in seeking integrative, natural, and even metaphysical healing modalities to provide the most nurturing of environments for my babies.

I had always believed in integrative and holistic approaches to wellness, so much so, once I got myself and my two kids into a better space, I started my company to help others.

Not that I typically quote clichés, but they say that necessity is the motherhood of invention.

So, I invented... a fabulously unique and powerful aroma-therapy series (Synergy Sprays) and while doing so, stepped fully into my role as the ultimate MAMA (Modern Alternative Mom Advocate).

Synergy Sprays are proprietary formulations of 4-5 pure, exceptional quality essential oils (per blend) designed to effect change, as is the case with all higher vibrational frequency, shammanistically rooted, eco-conscious oriented plant-based healing modalities, simultaneously on all three levels of your being: mind-body-spirit.

This is where my journey began... by admitting I had been brainwashed and stigma-stuck. Today, my company that started back in 2011, is scaling. Today, my book, *The ABCs of CBD: The Essential Guide*, has sold tens of thousands of copies — becoming one of the most respected and utilized resources across the Cannabis and hemp industries. I wrote it to explain "why pot is not what we were taught."

Though I've accomplished a lot, I also know this is just the beginning. We have much work yet to do and so much promise and potential to realize.

With legalization and decriminalization, we have a chance of correcting the errors of the past — where we allowed entire com-munities to be decimated by institutional racism (aka prohibition).

We have a chance at creating really great medical programs and educating practitioners beyond the old paradigms that excluded any information about the endocannabinoid receptor system, never mind the miracle of plants as whole food nutrition.

We have an opportunity to create a vibrant future by giving patients the right to grow or access medicine. Cannabis, and its cousin, hemp, actually work synergistically with our bodies and brains as opposed to creating fatal dependencies as we have seen with the (man-made) opiate epidemic designed not to treat common injuries, debilitating illnesses, and more, but to generate billions of dollars for manufacturers and Big Pharma.

We have a future that will allow us to expand research into modern-day explosions of issues like autism, Alzheimer's, and cancers.

We will be able to delve deeper into the promise of plant medicine and break down the miracles of not just the more famous cannabinoids, THC and CBD, but the other 138+ that we are only just beginning to discover.

To be a part of this moment in our culture and zeitgeist is exciting and challenging in ways I could not have imagined. Yet, I would not trade a single moment of it. This is my life, my mission, and my passion.

Shira Adler:
Author (*The ABCs of CBD*).
Speaker. Inspirer.
Founder & CEO

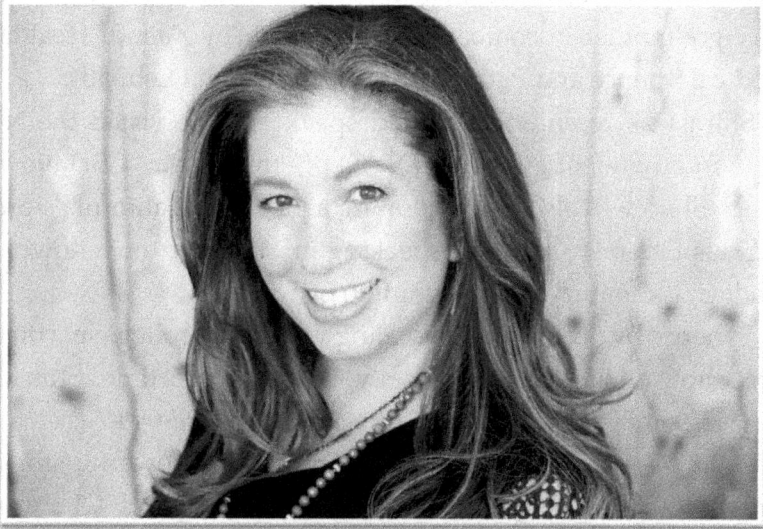

Author, Speaker, Inspirer — Shira Adler is a voice for our time, building from an eclectic background in spiritual care to her role over the last decade plus as a holistic media-wellness personality, CBD educator, advocate, activist, and entrepreneur.

Shira is Founder & CEO of Synergy by Shira Adler, a holistic media and wellness ComPASSIONate Care company that created the world's first (and only) CBD infused aromatherapy Synergy Spray part of a unique holistic regimen with full spectrum high mg tinctures and essential oil infused topicals.

Shira is the acclaimed author of *The ABCs of CBD™: The Essential Guide* and internationally recognized for her appearances on Bravo, GMA, The Today Show, and more. Reuters calls Shira "the Marijuana Mama" — and she is a contributor across myriad digital and linear platforms on topics ranging from holistic wellness, CBD, Cannabis and hemp industries, social activism and advocacy, and FemPowered entrepreneurism.

With high accolades by esteemed colleagues in the hemp and Cannabis industries, not to mention myriad media entities for her podcasts, appearances, and articles — Shira has been described as the "Mrs. Fields of Healing" and her new favorite: the "canna-fairy-godmother-in-combat-boots" coined by Vireo Health's Medical Science and Patient Liaison, Dr. Paloma Lehfeldt.

Shira was recently a featured speaker and assisted the NY Now international gift show (NYC) organize their "CBD Now" panel. Shira will also be moderating a panel for California's prestigious Emerald Cup, and speaking in Malta for the renowned Medical CannaBiz World Summit.

Synergy by Shira Adler is scaling with new strategic partners Greenhouse Ventures and finally, in her spare time, Shira is working on her second book *Pink Moccasins (And Other Footwear Inspired Tales Of Fempowerment)* — an array of powerful stories about women in the Cannabis and hemp industries—"because you can't walk in another woman's shoes, but you sure as hell can admire them."

Timothy Mount

Tell me about your journey with Cannabis/CBD. What is your area of expertise?

I first saw CBD in 2014, at a natural products trade show in Chicago. I remember thinking, "Isn't that stuff illegal?" Little did I know, I was seeing the first products on the market of what has turned out to be a tidal wave of CBD supplements over the years. Slowly, more and more companies popped up, but I didn't try CBD until 2016. My first experience was, well, unremarkable. It was a low dosage and very expensive at the time. I didn't continue taking it. However, I started to hear remarkable stories about hemp extract from colleagues and gave it another shot a year later.

I am a second-degree black belt in judo and have been practicing the sport for more than a decade. My body has taken a beating and the injuries have piled up. A day didn't go by when I wasn't in pain – mostly my neck from the whiplash of being thrown to the ground over and over. It hurt to turn my head and I suffered from chronic migraines. For anyone who has experienced a migraine, they can appreciate the fear of not knowing when the next excruciating episode would occur. I was desperate for anything that would help and CBD had gained a reputation for helping with chronic pain and migraines.

My next experience was miraculous. I tried a stronger dosage and felt relief almost instantly. I was hooked!

When did your interest start in Cannabis and why? Why did you start your business?

My background as a Certified Master Herbalist and Clinical Nutritionist, plus my work as a formulator and director of education for a large supplement company has me curious. What was going on? What's in this stuff? I dove into the research and read nearly everything I could get my hands on. Research was limited due to the gray area of legality at the time, but I found hundreds of testimonials online of similar experiences like the one I had.

My colleague and best friend, Jessica Mulligan, was also dealing with her own personal struggles. Not with pain like myself, but she had anxiety and insomnia that was affecting her daily life. It was heartbreaking to hear her describe feeling overwhelmed and seeing her on the verge of tears every day.

I remember the phone call clearly. Jess called me with an excitement in her voice I hadn't heard for a while. She'd tried CBD and was able to sleep through the night for the first time in eight months. Her anxiety was manageable and she felt like herself again. I couldn't believe it! How could one plant have so many benefits?

It was during that phone call that Jess and I first thought of the idea of starting our own CBD company. We both wanted to share the benefits we experienced with the world. People needed to know that there was help. We had been in key management positions for a large collagen brand and had always wanted to build our own brand of natural products. What better inspiration could there be than our combined personal experiences with CBD? We'd found our passion.

Still, there seemed to be a new CBD company every day, some good and some with questionable practices. We weren't sure we could survive as just another CBD brand. That's when Jess suggested we do one thing and do it better than anyone else – we wanted to be the best at what we did and not try to be everything to everyone. So, the decision was made (from Jess's astute observation) that we would focus on Women's Wellness and not just use CBD, but tailor our formulas with other female-specific nutrients to make comprehensive formulas to support the benefits women were looking for when taking CBD. Over and over, we heard the same answers from the women we spoke with, they needed help with mood and anxiety support, stress management and sleep improvement. **Winged** was born and our mission is to help the women of today's world catch their breath and harness the power of CBD and other nutrients so they can be the best version of themselves.

What are the misconceptions of Cannabis?

Hemp certainly carries the association of its illicit cousin marijuana. The most common reaction I get from consumers is that hemp will get them high or that taking a CBD supplement is similar to smoking a joint. Sometimes people will roll their eyes and say things like, "That stuff's not for me", as if I'm dealing drugs to them.

Hemp supplements have also come a long way since its initial legalization in 2014. Hemp was incredibly expensive to produce and often contained low doses at a high retail price. Hemp cultivars have also evolved to provide broader spectrum, more beneficial extracts. Because of this, someone might have tried a CBD supplement years ago, that had only a moderate benefit, unlike the higher quality supplement being produced today. I recommend everyone give it a second try.

The terminology of hemp supplements have also confused the public. There are products that are isolates, broad spectrum and full spectrum, but customers often don't know the difference. To clarify, isolates contain only CBD and no THC, but do not offer the "entourage effect" of other cannabinoids that many people swear by. Broad spectrum does contain many of the other cannabinoids beyond CBD (such as CBC, CBN, CBG, etc.) but has all of the THC removed from the product. This can be good and not so good because the process to completely remove THC may involve harsh solvents (ethanol, butane, propane) that leave a residual residue or other processing practices that alters the natural compounds of the "mother juice" extracted from the hemp plant.

This option is great for government employees or anyone concerned about THC showing up on a drug test, but still wants the benefit of the other cannabinoids. Full-Spectrum does contain trace amounts of THC, but is below the legal limit of 0.3% THC, so it meets the definition of hemp and not marijuana. That amount of THC is so low that there's no noticeable psychotropic effect (it won't get you high). Full-Spectrum products are often the cleanest, most beneficial products on the market because they retain much of their natural compounds from the hemp extract and don't require solvents for processing.

What questions are you most frequently asked?

Does it contain THC and will I fail a drug test?

Where and how is it grown? Is it grown in the USA and was it grown using organic farming practices?

What is the best dosage for someone to use? How does a new user start taking CBD and at what dosage?

What is the difference between CBD and hemp extract? Which one is indicated on the label? (Some companies label for "cannabinoids" that include more than just CBD and some label for CBD only on the front panel and indicate the total hemp extract on the back supplement facts panel.)

What does the dosage of oil (tincture) on the label mean? (Some companies put the total bottle content of CBD on the label while others indicate how much CBD per serving—total bottle content divided by the number of servings.) This is confusing because a consumer will say, "I take 600 mg," and they think that's how much is in each serving when they're only taking 20 mg CBD per serving and have a 30 day supply.

What questions should people be asking?

When companies have a QR Code on the back of their label, are they posting their actual lab results from a third-party independent lab, or is it a self-reported test on their own letterhead?

Customers should ask, "Why do I want to take CBD?" That's extremely important because CBD has so many benefits and may require different dosages to get the desired result. Pain management often requires a higher dose, but someone suffering from anxiety or sleep issues may not need nearly as much. Also, CBD isn't a magic cure-all! There are lots of other ingredients that may support the benefit someone is looking for. At Winged, we believe in developing comprehensive formulas that contain the correct dosage of CBD for each product based on the benefit someone is looking for, and then tailoring that formula to a woman's body that includes secondary nutrients to amplify the effect and deliver better benefits than CBD alone.

Give me a few examples of a positive experience, benefits, or success stories.

There are so many examples it's hard to choose just one. On a daily basis, we receive testimonials about how Winged products have changed someone's life. One particular moment comes to mind; it was the first time I saw what CBD could do for someone firsthand. We had just launched our Sleepy Gummies at a tradeshow. A woman approached our booth in an obviously frazzled state of mind. We began talking. She'd never tried CBD and seemed skeptical. She opened up to me about how stressful her work and personal life had been lately and how she hadn't slept well in years. She said she was constantly tired and her exhaustion made it hard to handle the stress of the day. She seemed desperate for relief. Since it was midday, I offered her a Sleepy Gummy and told her to take it before bed. The next day, the moment the show doors opened, she was the first one at our booth. She was ecstatic and had a glow about her that hadn't been there the day before. She got a full eight hours of sleep that night; the first time in as long as she could remember. She broke down in tears and gave me a long hug while thanking me. "This is the first time that I've had hope in a long time," she said. It really moved me how much a supplement could impact a person's life. It's these types of experiences that drive our company and fuel our passion because we know we're making a difference.

What is the recommended starting dose for clients? Can you overdose, and what are the side effects?

We recommend starting slow with 5 mg of CBD at first. See how your body reacts and gradually increase the dosage over time.

I don't know if "overdose" is the right term because it implies serious side effects or even death (like taking too much medication or illegal drugs). To my knowledge, those types of serious side effects have never occurred with a CBD supplement. I would say that as Americans, we think, "more is better," but for CBD, I don't believe that's the case. Mostly, I think people are throwing their money away by taking more than they need.

How has CBD helped you, clients, or others where other products were unsuccessful?

My personal ongoing experience with CBD comes mostly from pain management, stress handling, and sleep. When I was 20 years old, I was hit by a truck driving 45 mph, while on foot and nearly died. To this day, I suffer from the injuries I sustained. I also practiced judo, a rough martial art, for two decades until I retired from the sport because my body felt broken. I was worried that I'd be hobbled as an older adult and focused on healing my body naturally through a number of natural practices that include diet and supplementation, meditation, and exercise. CBD had been a big part of my recovery and my ability to enjoy life without the limitations of those injuries. I feel the most amount of comfort internally than I've felt in years.

As a co-founder of a supplement brand, stress is unavoidable. It's a good thing I sell a product that helps me calm my nerves! At night, my mind can race with a million different ideas and I've found it harder and harder to get a good night sleep. I'm a regular user of several of our Winged products, including our Balance Oil for comfort, Relaxation Gummies for on the spot stress handling, and Sleepy Gummies to help me fall asleep and get a good night of rest so I can be fresh and focus on the day at hand.

What changes in the industry do you foresee coming in the future? For legal issues as well as a consumer viewpoint.

The big unknown is how the FDA will impose regulations on the industry. When and what they do is anyone's guess.

As the public becomes more educated about CBD and hemp, I believe there will be more understanding about quality, dosage, and supporting ethical business practices. Unfortunately, there are some bad apples out there trying to make a quick buck on a hot product by cutting corners and making outrageous medical claims. We applaud the FDA and regulators for cracking down on this because the public should only be exposed to safe, high-quality products. I recommend customers purchase products certified by the U.S. Hemp Authority, which goes through a stringent auditing process to verify a company is meeting the highest and best standards of manufacturing and sales.

There are several exciting areas of research and development underway that may improve the current hemp extract market.

First, clinical research is underway on CBD and some other cannabinoids that we anticipate will validate many of the benefits consumers experience now. Innovation and delivery methods of CBD will also be fun to watch. Absorption, bioavailability and bioactivity of CBD is being looked at closely to ensure the products a person takes gets into the body easily and effectively. Plus, as government authorities develop a regulatory framework, we may see improved farming and extraction processes, easier access to cost-effective products, and a general acceptance of hemp as a safe, beneficial nutrient that doesn't carry today's stigmas.

What do you wish people knew or understood about CBD?

Just like different varieties of apples, there are different varieties of hemp plants. Some are better used for products that use its fibers or seeds, while other strands make more nutritious supplements. One variety of hemp may have a different cannabinoid profile than another. This means that not all products are equal, and as a consumer, it may not always be the least expensive option that offers the best benefits for that person.

What is important to look for when selecting a CBD product ?

Choosing a company certified by the U.S. Hemp Authority should be the first stop for a consumer so they know they're purchasing a quality product. Next, each company offers its own unique set of products. Which one is right for them? Do they prefer the convenience of soft gels, the delicious taste of gummies, or want to incorporate oils into recipes? At Winged, we specialize in women's needs when taking CBD and want to do it the best that we can by adding additional female-specific nutrients like evening primrose oil, black cohosh, vitex or lemon balm to customize our products to the Winged women who take them.

At Winged, we also believe in transparency and philanthropy. A customer should know exactly what is going into their body, be able to clearly understand the product label and have access to third-party testing using a QR code on the label. A customer should also believe in the mission of the company. At Winged, we're committed to supporting and empowering women and have partnered with a charity called MOST that mentors young women to fulfill their potential.

About Timothy Mount

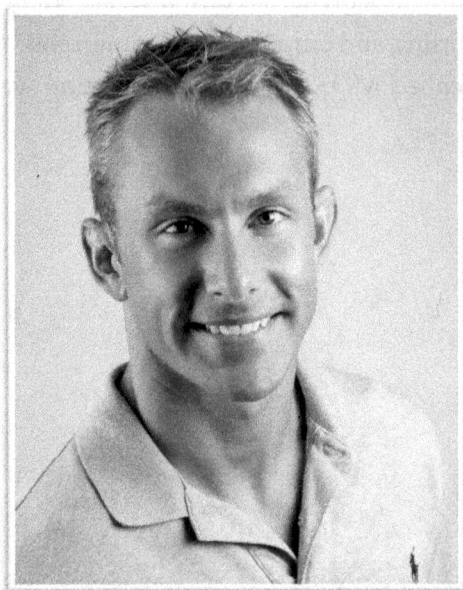

Timothy Mount is a Certified Clinical Nutritionist and Certified Master Herbalist and has presented at many of the leading natural health conventions and been featured on over 30 of the top natural health radio shows nationwide. Tim has worked as the Director of Education, Formulator, and Sales Manager for several leading brands in the natural products industry for over a decade. In 2018, he co-founded Winged Nutrition, a premium woman's wellness brand that focuses on comprehensive formulas that include CBD and other female-specific nutrient to help women in today's world be the best versions of themselves.

Wade Laughter

My first experience with Cannabis was in 1968. I was a summer camp counselor at a Boy Scout camp teaching swimming and boating. One afternoon, two scoutmasters invited me to go for a walk and we smoked a joint. It was lovely. However, I was an athlete hoping for a swimming scholarship and smoking seemed like a bad idea. Cannabis was very illegal and expensive so my use was intermittent. In 1976, I entered a spiritual community that required me to abstain from taking intoxicants. In 1984, I left the community with my twin daughters and their mother. My work life from 1984, until 1996, required me to pass random drug tests. So, from 1976, until 1996, I used very little Cannabis.

In 1995, I was diagnosed with glaucoma and the prescription medications given for glaucoma made me very ill. I explored all possible alternatives to those prescription meds and decided to learn about Cannabis. I quickly realized I would have to grow my own Cannabis if I wanted to know it was free of contamination. Since then, I have organized several patient collectives based on California's Proposition 215 and Senate Bill 420.

In 2008, we found and named the Cannabis cultivar known as Harlequin. She was one of the very first CBD-rich Cannabis plants that was available. From 2009, until 2015, cuttings of Harlequin were available at dispensaries in the San Francisco Bay area. Harlequin produces two to three times as much CBD as THC and is an excellent producer of Cannabis medicine and an excellent mother plant for breeding purposes. In 2010, I closed our warehouse operation and devoted several years to learning the science of Cannabis as medicine. In 2011, we left San Francisco and bought a small farm near Nevada City in California.

In 2014, I helped to create a product line of sublingual tinctures known as "Wonder Drops." The line was a low CBD high THC [1:25, a CBD and THC 2:1 and a high CBD low THC 25:1. This was a very successful line in the California dispensary market. All the Cannabis came from our farm and we were involved in the manufacturing and formulation of the products. In January of 2016, our local government passed a new law that prohibited commercial Cannabis activity in our county. This forced us to withdraw from the Wonder Drops project.

Also in January of 2016, I met a young father, Forrest Hurd, whose son suffers from epilepsy. His diagnosis is Lennox-Gastaut syndrome, which means he is subject to most forms of seizures. Forrest had tried various Cannabis products available in dispensaries to control his son's seizures at great cost and to little benefit. Then, he got some oil made from a cultivar named "Medi-Haze" that showed up in our garden in the summer of 2012. His son had 80+ seizures in the 24 hours before his first dose of Medi-Haze. After that first dose, he stopped seizing and by continuing to give him small doses on a regular schedule, he went four months with no seizures at all. The results we see are not usually that dramatic, but there are many stories like it. An interesting note here: This child needs CBD and THC to control his seizures and the ratio of cannabinoids needed for seizure control has changed over the last few years.

Forrest and I, along with the help of many in our community, created a charity, Caladrius Network, whose mission statement is "to provide education and, if appropriate, Cannabis therapies to the families of catastrophically ill children at no cost to those families, ever." Catastrophically ill is a specific medical term, which means the condition is typically fatal and our medicine has no effective treatment. By January of 2019, we were providing specific preparations for 146 families and had another 740 families in our intake process when state law changed again and made our activities illegal.

Most of these kids suffered from one of three conditions: untreatable cancers, epilepsy, and a genetic condition known as EB (epidermolysis bullosa). EB causes the proteins that help our skin bind to the underlying tissues to not form properly and this results in very fragile skin. Clothing can be enough to cause the skin to blister and slough off leaving raw wounds. Many of the EB kids die of sepsis or skin cancers. We tried to prepare enough medications to get our families through 2019, before our legal protections disappeared. In the current "legal" California marketplace, the preparations that helped these kids and many other folks are unavailable and/or very expensive.

Due to prohibition, there is so much fear and misinformation about Cannabis medicine that, it is hard to know where to start.

MISCONCEPTIONS INCLUDE (ALL of these are wrong):

- You have to get stoned
- There are only a couple of kinds of "weed" (indica, sativa, ruderalis, and hemp)
- CBD does get you high
- CBD is all you need and it cures everything
- You must decarboxylate Cannabis oil to make good products
- Hemp and Cannabis are different plants
- CBD is medical and THC is recreational
- If some is good, more is better
- The highest potency test results means the best/most desirable product.

I am often asked to help someone whose doctor has recommended they might try Cannabis for a certain condition or diagnosis. They come to me because they don't want to "get stoned" and they have heard that I know about that. We have found that, depending on the person, their condition, and their willingness or ability to follow directions, there is usually a way to help them find benefit without debilitating intoxication. The intent with Cannabis medicine is to work with the body and the endocannabinoid system.

There are many different ways of getting Cannabis medicine into the body and the effects vary widely. We always start with very small doses and increase the dose very slowly. We provide guidance to the end user on how to find the perfect dose for them. Every person is different, so I flinch when I hear someone giving blanket dosing guidelines for all users.

Humans seem to have extremely wide variation in sensitivity to Cannabis. There are likely many reasons for this but one is that some people may have only a few cannabinoid receptors (CB1) in their central nervous system (CNS). Others may have gross abundance of CB1 receptors in the CNS. The response to the same number of milligrams of THC in those two populations would be wildly different. The entire study of the endocannabinoid system is still a developing science.

There is a lot of interest in the healing potential of CBD from hemp. Remember that hemp and Cannabis are the same plant. My point of view is that all Cannabis has the potential to be "medical" Cannabis. If Cannabis is to be used in a therapeutic way, it must be free of any contamination from pesticides, fungicides, heavy metals, and pathological microorganisms. Because Cannabis is a bio accumulator, it will draw these materials from the environment in which it is grown. In California, Cannabis products must pass testing requirements that no food or drink could pass. Legal Cannabis in California is likely the cleanest consumer product available. Hemp products under most law is only tested for the amount of THC. There is very little testing to ensure quality, potency, or purity of hemp products. Some product makers test their material, but few of them test to the standards of Cannabis. The southern California chapter of Americans for Safe Access (ASA) sent a team out to buy CBD products at stores in the Los Angeles area. They bought a range of CBD products from several storefronts. They sent these samples for testing at an analytical lab looking at three criteria: contamination, potency (was there as much CBD in the product as stated), and the presence of more than 0.3% THC. Every single sample failed for one or more of these criteria. Most of the samples failed for more than one reason, and nine of the 20 failed on all counts. So, it is still very much a buyer beware situation in the hemp marketplace.

That being said, there are some farmers and manufacturers doing good work with hemp. It is helping to normalize Cannabis in our culture and provides cannabinoids to consumers.

An observation about hemp law: if hemp were to be defined as the Cannabis plant that produced less than a certain amount of all cannabinoids instead of being defined by THC levels, the law would make sense from a botanical science and a regulatory point of view. Because hemp is defined by THC levels, we have all kinds of people growing "CBDs" and trying to make products with no rules to protect public health and safety. In 2014, our production garden had five different versions of the Cannabis plant that could be called hemp, but we treated them as medicinal Cannabis plants for extraction.

One reason we had so many type 3 plants in the garden that year is because in 2013, I met my first catastrophically ill "kid." He was in a wheelchair and attended a Cannabis industry event with his family. His body was locked up in a condition known as "rictus". His fists were clenched, muscles locked up, and he had a painful grimace on his face. I spoke with his parents and learned he needed high CBD low THC oil (type 3) to help control his seizures. He was on 15 different anti-seizure medications and they were not working anymore. One of the side effects of those meds caused him to go blind. We gave the family plant material to make the oil they needed and looked for other plants with similar chemistry. In 2014, we found that a plant known as Remedy gave dramatic improvement in the frequency, intensity, and duration of his seizures. Today, he only requires one seizure medication, he is no longer blind, he no longer needs to wear a diaper, and he engages with the people around him. He responds really well to certain versions of Cannabis that could be called hemp; whereas others with a similar diagnosis, need Cannabis with THC and CBD to control their seizures. There is no one-size-fits-all in Cannabis medicine.

Most folks don't have as dire circumstances as I have described. I do believe that most of us in our culture are living through what Russo and others have referred to as "Cannabinoid Deficiency Syndromes." The idea here is that for a variety of reasons, our bodies are no longer producing the endocannabinoids we need to maintain health. These factors include food safety and quality, environmental toxins, stress, and lack of exercise. The reason Cannabis has such powerful effects in our bodies is because Cannabis makes compounds that mimic compounds our bodies make that are needed to regulate homeostasis.

In my experience, the real "magic" of Cannabis medicine happens when we can "identify the chemistry we want in the plants and then extract that chemistry intact as possible, put it into a product that an informed end user can benefit from." This means preserving all of the cannabinoids (neutral and acid forms) and terpenes. It means putting it into a dose able form that is palatable and repeatable. It means the end user knows how to find the dose that gives them the benefit they are seeking without undesirable side effects. We call that dose the "sweet spot." The end user has to be informed on how to know the path to arrive at the sweet spot.

People have asked me to explain CBD to them and I usually answer about some of the effects I have observed. I have never worked with isolated concentrates of CBD. Our experiences with crude homemade extractions were so good there was no reason to add to the cost or the chance of losing efficacy. The latest science suggests that old school crude with all kinds of cannabinoids and terpenes contributes to, what is termed, the "entourage effect" and seems to make the best medicine for most conditions. I wish more people understood this idea. In exactly the same way that Cannabis is not just about THC, it is also not just about CBD. There are approximately 160 cannabinoids that have been studied enough to be published in peer-reviewed science literature. I hear rumors from other countries of as many as 1000 being looked for in the plants. We are still learning how THC and CBD—two of the 160 published—work in our bodies.

If I could wave a magic wand, I would undo the last 70+ years since prohibition became federal in 1937. Imagine if science had spent those years studying this plant for the potential benefits to health. For its effects on cancer, on pain signaling, on autism, on IBS, on neuropathy, on MS, on memory, for traumatic brain injury, for agitation and anger in dementia, on autoimmune issues, for Huntington's, and not to forget, epilepsy. All of the suffering we might have avoided, all the costs of health care and the drug war. Look at how the drug war most heavily impacted only certain people in our culture. It would remove the stigma of multigenerational lies about a plant that can do no harm. All the criminality and alienation, the fear and anger, the killings that have happened. All of that is due to trying to enforce a prohibition that began on very shady grounds and ended up in a culture at war with itself.

All that harm over a healing and beautiful flowering plant that is easy to grow outdoors and is, in fact, full of potential medical benefit and, in my experience, is far less addictive than coffee.

About Wade Laughter

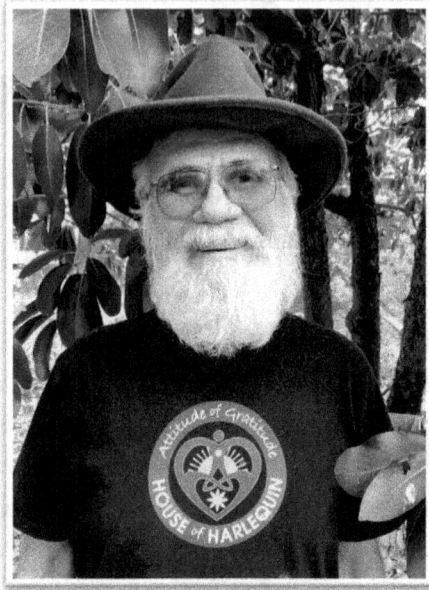

Wade Laughter's first professional work in agriculture began in 1974, after discharge from the U.S. Navy. Wade bought a 14-acre farm with his family to grow biodynamic and organic berries. Berry farming was too much work for too little money. In 1976, Wade entered a spiritual community where he spent eight years as a teacher of community spiritual practices as well as building teams to accomplish various projects for the community. In 1978, Wade was blessed with twin daughters who attended Waldorf School for their primary and secondary education. From 1976, to 1995, Wade engaged in little to no Cannabis use.

In 1986, Wade moved to San Francisco where he stayed until 2010. In 1995, a diagnosis of severe glaucoma and complications from prescribed medications to treat glaucoma led Wade to Cannabis as medicine. The wide variety and quality of Cannabis available made him realize he would need to grow on his own in order to ensure a clean Cannabis supply. Living in San Francisco required Wade to learn about indoor cultivation starting in a closet and then in a garage. Wade found like-minded people who had need for Cannabis as medicine and ended up in a small warehouse in South of Market in San Francisco. The patients formed a collective and surplus medicine, beyond the needs of the patient group, was sold to various dispensaries in the Bay Area and Southern California. During this time, Wade worked with many different cultivars; best known for "Strawberries", "Genius,"" Bubba Kush," and "Lemon Kush."

In 2007, Wade was fortunate enough to discover and name the cultivar known as "Harlequin," one of the first CBD-rich cultivars to gain recognition. When Wade realized its importance, the collective began to give it away to as many people as possible for a number of years. Since Wade's discovery and the dissemination of Harlequin, he has worked with clinicians, researchers, Cannabis professionals, and patients. The work since then is finding new cultivars of interest to address the need of true medical benefit from Cannabis.

In 2011, Wade and his wife bought a beautiful 4-acre farm where he discovered the ease, beauty, and quality available in Cannabis done to the standards of medicine and regenerative practices. Wade then went on, in 2014, to develop and release the product known as "Wonder Drops" available in dispensaries across California. Wade was forced to withdraw from this business in 2016, when county supervisors passed an ordinance forbidding Cannabis business activity.

Wade's current project, House of Harlequin, was formed in 2015, as a not-for-profit mutual benefits corporation. In 2016, he joined with Forrest Hurd to found the Caladrius Network. Our mission statement: "To provide education, and if appropriate, Cannabis therapies to the families of catastrophically ill children at no cost to those families, ever." By January of 2019, we were actively supporting 146 children, and another 700 families were in our intake process. Before changes in California law forced us to shut down, we had given away more than $1.2 million in specific formulas. None of these patients "smoke" their medicine.

The House of Harlequin farm joined the Dragonfly Earth Medicine (DEM Pure) family of farms in 2017. As of 2019, local ordinance mandates no commercial Cannabis activity on Wade's farm, and for that reason, he has become an educator on regenerative farming practices and Cannabis as medicine. Wade summarizes his approach to Cannabis as medicine this way, "We find the chemistry profile needed in the Cannabis plant, capture and concentrate that profile, and preserve it in formulations that are appropriate for an educated end user so that they may consume it for their benefit."

Wade continues to work as an educator for local dispensaries and community groups seeking to learn about Cannabis cultivation and safe Cannabis use. He is active with numerous statewide Cannabis advocacy organization in Northern California and consults with local licensed Cannabis farms looking to use optimal cultivation practices. He is also working with Dragonfly Wellness, a vertically integrated locally owned pharmacy in Salt Lake City, Utah.

LEGAL

Michael J. Correia

Tell me about your journey with Cannabis, what is your area of expertise?

My journey with Cannabis began in 2013, when I became the first full-time Cannabis industry lobbyist. My expertise is in understanding the political process and being able to navigate an illegal, nascent Cannabis industry through Capitol Hill. I have spent years increasing the visibility of our industry and gathering support with politicians in Washington, D.C.

When did your interest start in Cannabis and why?

Although I smoked marijuana in high school and believed the war on drugs was a complete waste of time and money, it wasn't until Colorado and Washington passed legalization initiatives in 2012, that I became interested in this issue. It touches on so many policy issues: healthcare, criminal justice reform, racial equality, and federalism, I had to be part of it. It's the next great social policy issue of the 21st century.

What are the misconceptions of Cannabis?

One of the biggest misconceptions surrounding Cannabis is the stoner stereotype. The stereotype that "normal" people don't consume Cannabis. The stereotype is that if you consume Cannabis, you are a loser with no initiative, sitting in your parent's basement. There are many frequent consumers of Cannabis who are high functioning, as well as many infrequent consumers of Cannabis, who just want an occasional fun experience.

What are the five frequently asked questions on your topic?

1. Do you have samples?
2. What are your priorities?
3. What are the next states to legalize?
4. Who opposes you on Capitol Hill?
5. What companies should I invest in?
6. Bonus. When will Cannabis be legal?

What are the five questions people should be asking?

1. What does the movement need to achieve a successful outcome?
2. Is incremental reform more important that full legalization?
3. How do I get more involved?
4. Why are drug reform groups slowing up legalization?
5. What states should lobbying prioritize?

Give me a few examples of a positive experience, benefits, or success stories.

Most of my positive experiences come from politicians slowly changing their tunes and accepting Cannabis reform as the smart path forward. The satisfaction is not immediate, but still important and positive.

Give me an example of how Cannabis was life changing for someone you know.

Just being able to know that a family with a sick child is able to have access to potential medicine. That is always life changing and keeps me motivated.

How has Cannabis helped you or your clients where other products were unsuccessful?

I hear lots of stories from friends about being able to sleep better, be less anxious, deal with nagging pains, use fewer prescription drugs, etc.... all because of Cannabis.

What changes in the industry do you foresee coming in the future?

I see the professionalization of the industry when it comes to testing, labeling, product safety, etc. I see old-school legacy operators being pushed to the side as new investors and corporate operators start moving in.

What do you wish people knew or understood about Cannabis?

Although it is a drug and should be treated with respect, it is a lot safer (from a policy perspective) than alcohol, gambling, fast food, video games, etc. It should be judged accordingly and people should have an adult conversation about it.

Are there any questions that you feel you would like to address that were not asked?

No, this is thorough.

Can you discuss the legal issues that you are faced with working in the Cannabis industry?

The gray area that exists between state and federal conflict has always been a concern for people working in the Cannabis industry. As states moved forward, favorable American support grows, and the industry continues to grow; this is confusing. Congress needs to act to address prohibition for the safety of Cannabis industry employees.

What are your feelings regarding the social justice piece of this? There are still people in jail that should be released.

The War on Drugs and prohibition have ruined peoples' lives. As we move forward with Cannabis reform, we must include comprehensive language regarding restorative justice.

Can you explain the differences between state and federal issues?

The states are moving forward with legalization efforts. Their priorities focus on regulations and how a legal industry should operate. The federal government is still debating the merits of legalization....and it will take years to solve. The states are miles ahead of the federal government.

Can you explain the differences in the laws between CBD and THC?

That is a tricky question because CBD (derived from marijuana) is illegal. CBD (derived from hemp) is legal. And, consumers don't know the difference and many unsavory actors will take advantage of consumer ignorance and sell products that are not as advertised. A lot of policy issues need to be addressed to correct this. The simplest solution is amending the Controlled Substances Act and legalizing all Cannabis derived products.

What are current issues for the general public to understand?

The current issues for the general public to understand are that state Cannabis businesses cannot function like other legal businesses. There is a lack of access to financial institutions, the 280E tax provision, lack of federal research available, etc.

Can you please explain the difficulties people in the industry face because of the federal laws?

Not having access to banking services is a big challenge for businesses and consumers, who have to do transactions in cash.

Not being able to write off standard business deductions on your federal tax returns is hurting small businesses' ability to compete and survive. Not being able to research this plant, has slowed down, not up, the progress by decades....

Michael J. Correia
Director of Government Relations

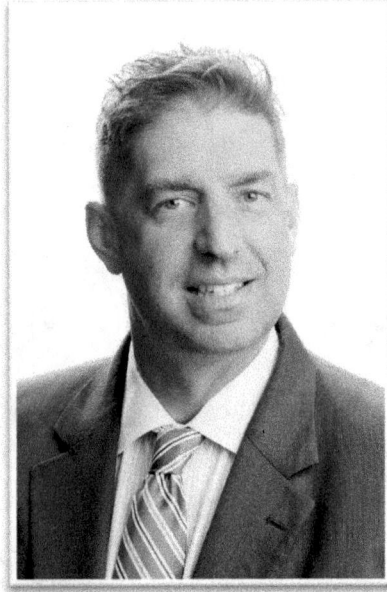

Michael Correia is director of government relations for the National Cannabis Industry Association. His focus is raising awareness and building support for the Cannabis industry's issues on Capitol Hill.

In addition, Michael works with other national organizations to increase the Cannabis industry profile nationally. Prior to joining NCIA, Michael spent many years working on Capitol Hill, including working for Rep. George Radanovich (R-CA), who retired in 2010, and the House Committee on Resources, serving three different Chairmen.

Previously, he was director of federal affairs for the American Legislative Exchange Council (ALEC) and senior project manager for the Committee for a Responsible Federal Budget. In both positions, he advocated for policies in Congress.

A campaign veteran, he has worked and volunteered on numerous political campaigns at the local, state, and federal levels over the past two decades. Michael is a graduate of the University of California, San Diego. A native of San Diego, he resides in Washington, D.C.

Rod Kight

Tell me about your journey with Cannabis.

I smoked Cannabis for the first time while in college and immediately loved it. I have always believed that it should be lawful. That being said, I did not consider it "medicine" until I used it in my mid-30s during chemotherapy treatments for testicular cancer. (I am 10 years in remission).

At first, I didn't try Cannabis as a medical aid, due to a misplaced belief that doing so would really be nothing more than using my illness it as an excuse to get high. However, on a particularly difficult day when I was feeling miserable, I broke down and smoked marijuana with my brother. The experience was stunning and remarkable. Within 15 minutes, I felt significantly better. For the first time in days, I had an appetite. My flu-like aches subsided and my nausea disappeared.

Certainly, I wasn't 100% better. However, I felt well enough to spend a pleasant evening talking with my brother. I ate two helpings of spicy Indian food and slept well enough to regain some lost energy. Had I not smoked marijuana that evening, I would have stayed in bed, not eaten, and spent most of the night tossing and turning, nauseated, and in agony. My energy levels would have continued their steep decline and I would have been worse off for the next treatment.

Cannabis helped me through chemotherapy, and I resolved at that time to become an advocate for its legalization. In addition to aiding with side effects of chemotherapy, new research suggests that it may also be important in the treatment and even prevention of certain diseases, including some forms of cancer.

What is your area of expertise?

I am an attorney who represents Cannabis businesses. In addition to usual business law matters pertinent to companies in any industry (drafting and negotiating contracts, forming and dissolving companies, protecting intellectual property, etc.), I provide in-depth consulting on compliance and strategic planning in the Cannabis industry. My firm focuses on hemp and CBD, and represents some of the largest and best hemp/CBD companies in the USA and the world. I speak at legal, business, and medical conferences, write articles, give interviews to media outlets, and advocate for Cannabis, both in the USA and internationally.

When did your interest in Cannabis start and why?

As a freshman in college, one of my hall mates brought some marijuana to school from his home. Several of us went into the woods to smoke it. I remember the giddy, time-traveling, and exhilarating experience as if it was yesterday. (To be clear, it was many decades from "yesterday"!) I am a musician and have always enjoyed listening and playing music with Cannabis. It relaxes me and opens up creative channels. Additionally, now that there is ample evidence of its medical utility, I also enjoy it for its health benefits. Although I enjoy a good glass of beer, wine, or whiskey, I find that I rarely drink to excess when I use Cannabis.

What are the misconceptions of Cannabis?

Unfortunately, the number of misconceptions about Cannabis appear to be countless. The primary ones I hear are that it is dangerous, a gateway drug, and that it promotes a lifestyle that is not congruent with being a good citizen, employee, or parent. In fact, none of these things are true. Additionally, as a business attorney, I encounter lots of people who think it is "green gold."

While Cannabis is, and has always been, a revenue-generating commodity, I believe that we are definitely seeing a "green rush" that will result in some business and financial failures. This is already beginning to occur.

What are the questions you are most frequently asked about Cannabis?

Is CBD legal?

The legal status of hemp depends on a number of factors. When derived from hemp, it is not a controlled substance. However, the FDA and many states contend that it cannot be used as a food ingredient or marketed as a dietary supplement and no medical claims can be made about it. Additionally, individual state laws impact the legal status of CBD within their borders.

Can I mail hemp and CBD?

Yes. The USPS recently lost a federal court case on this issue and the USDA has confirmed that interstate transport of hemp and hemp products, including via mail, is lawful. To be clear, it is completely lawful to mail hemp and hemp products, including CBD derived from hemp.

Can I ship hemp and CBD internationally?

It depends. If these things are lawful in the destination country, the answer is "yes". If not, the answer is "no."

Is hemp extract containing more than 0.3% THC legal?

This is an unresolved question of law. I have worked with clients on this issue, but there are no solid answers. Unfortunately, to date, both of the primary federal agencies that regulate hemp have failed to address it.

Does "total THC" count in measuring delta-9 THC concentrations for hemp?

It depends. According to the USDA's interim final rule regarding hemp production, a pre-harvest hemp plant's "total THC," which includes both delta-9 THC THCA, must be taken into account to determine whether it is lawful. However, this standard does not necessarily apply to post-harvested hemp, though there are a number of exceptions and unresolved issues regarding total THC in contexts other than pre-harvest testing.

What questions should people be asking?

Listed below are some questions Cannabis consumers and business owners should be asking.

Can I make medical claims about my CBD products? No. The FDA has stated that the Food, Drug & Cosmetic Act (FDCA) prohibits medical claims about CBD. This is based on its approval of a CBD based anti-seizure drug called Epidiolex and the FDAC's prohibition on making medical claims about compounds that have been the subject of clinical trials prior to those compounds being marketed in food or as dietary supplements. The FDA contends that CBD was not marketed prior to the Epidiolex trials and thus cannot be a food ingredient or marketed as a dietary supplement. I expect this position to change, either by FDA, or Congressional action.

Should I be using a hemp extract rather than CBD isolate?

It depends on a number of factors. However, currently (this was written in March, 2020) there is a better legal argument for using hemp extract than CBD isolate in formulations intended for ingestion.

What is the next big thing in Cannabis?

I think it is the emergence of so-called "novel cannabinoids" into the marketplace and in clinical trials, which include delta-8 THC, CBG, CBN, THCV, and CBC. Each has its own chemical and potential medical properties.

Should I be considering entering the international market?

Possibly. The U.S. market is far from saturated; however, there is heavy competition and the likelihood of a significant adjustment when multinational corporations enter the industry in earnest. By and large, the international market is not as developed as the U.S. market, thus leading to opportunities. That being said, there are a number of legal and logistical hurdles involved in operating an international Cannabis business. The most notable is the European Union's (EU) current prohibition on the use of CBD in food based on its Novel Food legislation. In order to add CBD to food the producer must first apply and obtain approval from the EU to do so. This process is expensive and time-consuming.

What can I do to help promote Cannabis legalization?

Educate your legislators.

Give me a few examples of a positive experience, benefits, or success stories.

I have so many positive stories. I have clients whose epileptic children have weaned off of powerful prescription medications by using Cannabis. Others have weaned themselves and/or their family members off of harmful and addictive drugs through Cannabis. And I've seen small businesses that have flourished in the new Cannabis industry. Many of my clients who started small a few years ago, often with home-based businesses, now have multi-million-dollar companies.

Give me an example of how Cannabis was life-changing for someone you know.

Cannabis changed my life! (See above.) I beat cancer, found a true calling, and am happier, more satisfied, and more financially successful than I have ever been. My story is not unusual.

What changes in the industry do you foresee coming in the future?

I see a large "reckoning" in the form of market consolidation, a drop in prices across the board, accompanied by wider acceptance of Cannabis by consumers and government officials throughout the USA and the world.

What do you wish people knew or understood about Cannabis?

Where do I start? Actually, the simplest and most straightforward thing I can propose is an understanding that hemp and marijuana are two forms of the same plant. Both are "Cannabis." The sole distinction is the concentrations of delta-9 THC: hemp has no more than 0.3% and marijuana has more than 0.3%. The term "Cannabis" is widely used, particularly on the west coast, as a synonym for "marijuana." However, and with a few exceptions, "Cannabis" is a botanical term. The legal terms of art are "marijuana" and "hemp."

What are your feelings regarding the social justice piece of this? There are still people in jail that should be released.

Social justice is arguably the top issue regarding Cannabis. I am passionate about this issue. Not only should Cannabis never have been deemed a controlled substance in the first place, but the difference in the way marijuana laws have been enforced between white and affluent people and poor people and people of color is grotesquely out of proportion. Anyone in jail for marijuana sale and/or use should be released immediately and their criminal records with respect to marijuana crimes expunged.

Can you explain the differences between state and federal issues?

The interplay between state and federal laws is called "federalism." Although federal law usually preempts contrary state law, a number of factors are involved in the enforceability of state and federal laws when they are in conflict. (Entire law school courses cover federalism!). With respect to marijuana, federal law is clear. It is illegal. However, more than half of the states have enacted laws legalizing it in some form. To a degree, and with some significant exceptions, the federal authorities have generally not enforced federal marijuana laws with respect to companies that are compliant with state law. Additionally, in several consecutive budget provisions, Congress has indicated that no federal funds can be used to interfere with medical marijuana activities that are legal at the state level. This federal-state conflict has created many, and perhaps most, of the obstacles and difficulties we now encounter with marijuana, from banking to interstate commerce to medical research to criminal and tax liability.

With respect to hemp and CBD, the federalism issue is somewhat reversed. Hemp is unequivocally lawful at the federal level. However, a number of states have enacted laws and regulations purporting to make hemp, or some forms of it, illegal. Whether federal law preempts (i.e., overrides) these state laws is a subtle issue that may take years to resolve. While I believe that federal law will control in most respects, we currently can only speculate at how the federalism issues will play out with respect to hemp and CBD.

Can you explain the differences in the laws between CBD and THC?

Whether CBD and THC are controlled substances (i.e., illegal drugs), they are lawful or not based on their source. Additionally, with respect to THC, it depends on its concentration. CBD and THC derived from hemp are lawful. The concentration of CBD from hemp is irrelevant. Any amount is lawful. However, THC from hemp in concentrations that do not exceed 0.3% is lawful. From the standpoint of the FDCA as regulated by the FDA, these compounds cannot be used as food ingredients or marketed as dietary supplements and no medical claims can be made about them. (This includes medical claims that are true and based on clinical research.) Generally speaking, this is based on the fact that both CBD and THC are the primary compounds in FDA approved drugs. As I mentioned above, the FDA is currently considering revising this position to allow CBD.

What would you tell a person just getting introduced to CBD products from a legal perspective as well as a manufacturing one? There are some bad products out there; how do people protect themselves?

As a manufacturer, there are a number of legal considerations such as using good manufacturing practices (I mean that as a legal term of art, which is often referred to as "GMP"), proper labeling, compliance with federal and state laws regarding the legal status of these products, etc. Much of my law practice involves advising manufacturers of hemp/CBD products, and I could write an entire book on that subject alone.

Consumers should first educate themselves about CBD and how it interacts with the endocannabinoid system. There are a number of reputable books and websites on the subject. Once you have a solid understanding of CBD, I recommend utilizing all of the standard ways for vetting products, including customer reviews, the company's website, reading the ingredient list (including laboratory certificates of analysis), and even calling and talking with the company from which you may buy a CBD product. If you have any question regarding a company's legal compliance and/or the quality of its product, move on. There are a large number of companies doing the right thing. Consequently, there are legitimate, easy to vet products on the market.

Rod Kight

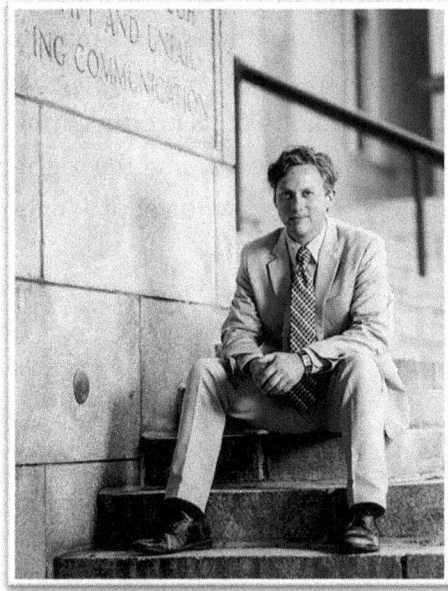

Rod is a Cannabis business law attorney who lives in Asheville, NC. He represents legal Cannabis businesses through-out the world and is editor and chief writer of the Kight On Cannabis law blog (www.kightonCannabis.com), a popular blog that discusses evolving legal issues affecting the Cannabis industry.

Rod is the author of *Cannabis Business Law: What You Need to Know*, published by Aspatore Books, a Thomson Reuters (WestLaw) Company, in August 2015. Rod is on the advisory board for the American Journal of Endocannabinoid Medicine (AJEM), for which he also writes a legal column. AJEM is the first printed, peer-reviewed medical Cannabis journal in North America.

Rod is frequently interviewed on Cannabis matters by major media outlets and has been quoted in the Wall Street Journal, Time, Business Insider, and Business Insurance. Additionally,

Rod has been listed in MG Magazine's list of "30 Powerful Litigators," Hemp Connoisseur Magazine's list of "100 People You Should Know," and High Time's "2020 Leaders in Cannabis Law."

A strong believer in Cannabis for personal and medical use after using it successfully during chemotherapy treatments for cancer (he is in remission), Rod is an attorney advocate for NORML. He is also a member of the International Cannabis Bar Association, the National Cannabis Industry Association, Women Grow, the Hemp Industries Association, and the North Carolina Industrial Hemp Association. Rod has been a presenter on Cannabis legal issues at seminars across the country. He has also drafted and presented Cannabis legislation to a foreign head of state.

Rod is married to his elementary school sweetheart, Ashley, who is also his office manager. Together they have five children. Rod is an avid musician who plays guitar in an Asheville-based rock band.

Conclusion

Cannabis has a seedy – ha, ha – reputation. In the past century, it has been something that is done underground or behind closed doors. It makes you think of shady deals and illegal behavior. It's something that stoners and criminals use, not people like you.

The proliferation of CBD stores and products have done a little bit to resuscitate its reputation, but it still somehow feels like something you can't talk about in polite society. If you've read this book, you know that's ridiculous. There should be no shame in using a product that is perfectly legal and scientifically proven to work.

Your body has an endocannabinoid system. Your body needs endocannabinoids to function properly. CBD doesn't introduce anything to your body that isn't already there. It stimulates your endocannabinoid system to work as it was designed to work. It doesn't get you high; it doesn't alter your mind in any way. Instead, it can help reduce pain and anxiety and ensure the proper functioning of your body's systems in general.

This book talked a lot about the versatility of the Cannabis plant. I wanted to provide you with accurate information from experts about the benefits of the plant and debunk the myths about CBD.

Hopefully, this book has taught you something. My goal was to teach you what Cannabis is, aside from its reputation. I wanted to tell you how it works in a very scientific way. This isn't a snake oil cure-all; this is a chemical that your body produces to keep itself in balance. As you age, your body produces less of it, so why not assist your body by introducing more to keep everything in balance?

I also wanted to help you weed – ha, ha – through the various types of products available. Are edibles right for you? Vaping? Oils? Balms? This book should give you the foundation to know the various pros and cons of the different products for the different conditions you are trying to treat.

And, perhaps most importantly, I wanted to help you learn how to maintain quality control. Not everyone is honest. Some unscrupulous vendors are willing to slap a label on anything and call it a CBD product. Hopefully, this book has taught you how to read a product's label to see what you are actually getting.

The average CBD customer faces a world of difficulty getting good information and quality products. Novelty products with no medicinal value, found with labels that look a lot like the products that will really help you, can be found at gas stations and convenience stores. Maybe it will be CBD, and maybe it won't be. How can you know?

Cannabidiol derived from hemp is now legal in all 50 states. That's a good thing! That will help make CBD more mainstream and available. Hopefully, more research will emerge and quality control standards will intensify.

In order to do that, I interviewed 31 experts from scientists, neurologists, nurses, doctors, to veterinarians, and a whole host of other people who have real-world experience working with Cannabis. They've shared their experiences working with this miracle drug. They've told you what they know. I've told you what I know.

And, we've only just started to scratch the surface. This was a difficult book to write because so much of the science is new. Just when I thought we were ready to go to press, I'd learn something new and I'd have to add some new information. It's hard to write a scientifically accurate book when the scientific body of knowledge keeps expanding.

Don't be afraid to do your own research and gather as much information as you can. You need to gauge whether taking CBD and in what dose is right for you. Do you want to take it before a workout? Do you want to take it to help with insomnia or anxiety? Do your research.

Don't buy into the fearmongering. The World Health Organization[6] says that CBD is generally well tolerated and has a good safety profile. The worst side effects tend to be loss of appetite, diarrhea, and dry mouth, and only a few experience those. Most effects can be managed by adjusting your dose.

That's it. I've taught you everything I know. Until I learn more, that is.

XOXO,
Doc Cynthia

---

[6] https://www.who.int/medicines/access/controlled-substances/5.2_CBD.pdf

www.ingramcontent.com/pod-product-compliance
Lightning Source LLC
Chambersburg PA
CBHW060833280326
41934CB00007B/770